# Synthesis Lectures on Biomedical Engineering

This series consists of concise books on advanced and state-of-the-art topics that span the field of biomedical engineering. Each Lecture covers the fundamental principles in a unified manner, develops underlying concepts needed for sequential material, and progresses to more advanced topics and design. The authors selected to write the Lectures are leading experts on the subject who have extensive background in theory, application, and design. The series is designed to meet the demands of the 21st century technology and the rapid advancements in the all-encompassing field of biomedical engineering.

Sudip Mukherjee · Vijay Sagar Madamsetty ·
Rakesh Chandra Reddy · Lipi Pradhan ·
Devyani Yenurkar · Sumit Manna ·
Durba Banerjee

# Nanocrystals in Cancer Theranostics

Recent Developments

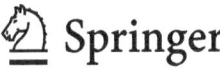

Sudip Mukherjee
School of Biomedical Engineering
Indian Institute of Technology
Varanasi, Uttar Pradesh, India

Rakesh Chandra Reddy
Immuneel Therapeutics Private Limited
Bengaluru, Karnataka, India

Devyani Yenurkar
School of Biomedical Engineering
Indian Institute of Technology
Varanasi, Uttar Pradesh, India

Durba Banerjee
School of Biomedical Engineering
Indian Institute of Technology
Varanasi, Uttar Pradesh, India

Vijay Sagar Madamsetty
Polyrna Therapeutics
Cambridge, MA, USA

Lipi Pradhan
School of Biomedical Engineering
Indian Institute of Technology
Varanasi, Uttar Pradesh, India

Sumit Manna
School of Biomedical Engineering
Indian Institute of Technology
Varanasi, Uttar Pradesh, India

ISSN 1930-0328  ISSN 1930-0336 (electronic)
Synthesis Lectures on Biomedical Engineering
ISBN 978-3-032-04132-6  ISBN 978-3-032-04133-3 (eBook)
https://doi.org/10.1007/978-3-032-04133-3

© The Editor(s) (if applicable) and The Author(s), under exclusive license to Springer Nature Switzerland AG 2026

This work is subject to copyright. All rights are solely and exclusively licensed by the Publisher, whether the whole or part of the material is concerned, specifically the rights of translation, reprinting, reuse of illustrations, recitation, broadcasting, reproduction on microfilms or in any other physical way, and transmission or information storage and retrieval, electronic adaptation, computer software, or by similar or dissimilar methodology now known or hereafter developed.

The use of general descriptive names, registered names, trademarks, service marks, etc. in this publication does not imply, even in the absence of a specific statement, that such names are exempt from the relevant protective laws and regulations and therefore free for general use.

The publisher, the authors and the editors are safe to assume that the advice and information in this book are believed to be true and accurate at the date of publication. Neither the publisher nor the authors or the editors give a warranty, expressed or implied, with respect to the material contained herein or for any errors or omissions that may have been made. The publisher remains neutral with regard to jurisdictional claims in published maps and institutional affiliations.

This Springer imprint is published by the registered company Springer Nature Switzerland AG
The registered company address is: Gewerbestrasse 11, 6330 Cham, Switzerland

If disposing of this product, please recycle the paper.

# Contents

| | | | |
|---|---|---|---|
| **1** | **Introduction** | | 1 |
| 1.1 | What Are Nanocrystals? | | 3 |
| | 1.1.1 | Organic Nanocrystals | 4 |
| | 1.1.2 | Inorganic Nanocrystals | 4 |
| | 1.1.3 | Hybrid Nanocrystals | 4 |
| 1.2 | Functional Properties of Nanocrystals | | 4 |
| | 1.2.1 | Organic Nanocrystals | 4 |
| | 1.2.2 | Inorganic Nanocrystals | 5 |
| | 1.2.3 | Hybrid Nanocrystals | 5 |
| 1.3 | Biocompatibility and Toxicity | | 6 |
| | 1.3.1 | Organic Nanocrystals | 6 |
| | 1.3.2 | Inorganic Nanocrystals | 6 |
| 1.4 | Synthesis and Applications of Nanocrystals | | 7 |
| | 1.4.1 | Synthesis of Organic Nanocrystals | 7 |
| | 1.4.2 | Synthesis of Inorganic Nanocrystals | 7 |
| 1.5 | Therapeutic Applications and Mechanisms | | 8 |
| | 1.5.1 | Enhanced Drug Delivery and Tumor Targeting | 8 |
| | 1.5.2 | Controlled Drug Release | 8 |
| | 1.5.3 | Overcoming Multidrug Resistance | 9 |
| | 1.5.4 | Radiotherapy Enhancement | 9 |
| | 1.5.5 | Immunomodulation and Combination Therapies | 9 |
| | 1.5.6 | Reduced Systemic Toxicity | 9 |
| 1.6 | Translational Challenges and Clinical Outlook | | 10 |
| 1.7 | Scope of This Book | | 10 |
| 1.8 | Structure of This Book | | 10 |
| 1.9 | Conclusion | | 11 |
| References | | | 11 |

| | | |
|---|---|---|
| **2** | **Types of Nanocrystals, Synthesis and Properties: Organic Nanocrystals, Inorganic Nanocrystals, Hybrid Nanocrystals** ......................... | 21 |
| | 2.1  Organic Nanocrystals ............................................... | 22 |
| | 2.2  Inorganic Nanocrystals ............................................. | 25 |
| | 2.3  Hybrid Nanocrystals ............................................... | 29 |
| | References ............................................................... | 38 |
| **3** | **Nanocrystals Applications in Cancer Therapy** ......................... | 41 |
| | 3.1  Introduction ....................................................... | 41 |
| | 3.2  Types of Nanocrystals ............................................. | 44 |
| |     3.2.1  Organic Nanocrystals ....................................... | 44 |
| |     3.2.2  Inorganic Nanocrystals ..................................... | 45 |
| |     3.2.3  Hybrid Nanocrystals ....................................... | 45 |
| |     3.2.4  Lipid-Based Nanocrystals .................................. | 48 |
| | 3.3  Inorganic Nanocrystals ............................................ | 50 |
| |     3.3.1  Photothermal and Photodynamic Therapy .................... | 55 |
| |     3.3.2  Photothermal Therapy (PTT) ............................... | 55 |
| |     3.3.3  Photodynamic Therapy (PDT) .............................. | 55 |
| |     3.3.4  Combination with Drug Delivery ........................... | 56 |
| |     3.3.5  Magnetic Manipulation .................................... | 56 |
| | 3.4  Nanocrystals as Anticancer Agents ................................. | 58 |
| |     3.4.1  Radiosensitizers ........................................... | 59 |
| |     3.4.2  Direct Cytotoxicity ........................................ | 59 |
| |     3.4.3  Combination Therapies .................................... | 60 |
| | References ............................................................... | 61 |
| **4** | **Immunomodulation, Immunotherapy, Biotherapeutics Through Nanocrystals** .......................................................... | 69 |
| | 4.1  Design Principles of Nanocrystal Formulations ..................... | 70 |
| | 4.2  Nanocrystal-Mediated Delivery of Immunomodulators and Biotherapeutics ............................................... | 71 |
| | 4.3  Theranostic Integration: Imaging-Guided Immune Activation ......... | 72 |
| |     4.3.1  Diagnostic Component ..................................... | 72 |
| |     4.3.2  Therapeutic Component .................................... | 72 |
| | 4.4  Preclinical Applications of Theranostic Nanocrystals ................ | 74 |
| | References ............................................................... | 77 |
| **5** | **Radiotherapeutics Applications of Nanocrystals: PTT, PDT** ............ | 85 |
| | 5.1  Fundamentals of Photothermal Therapy with Nanocrystals ............ | 87 |
| |     5.1.1  Material Innovations: Gold, Copper Chalcogenides, and Tantalum-Based Nanocrystals ......................... | 88 |
| |     5.1.2  Tumour Targeting and the Enhanced Permeability and Retention (EPR) Effect ............................... | 91 |

|   |   | 5.1.3 | Photothermal-Induced Modulation of the Tumour Microenvironment | 95 |
|---|---|---|---|---|
|   | 5.2 | | Principles and Mechanisms of Photodynamic Therapy with Nanocrystals | 96 |
|   |   | 5.2.1 | Nanocrystal Platforms for Enhanced Photosensitizer Delivery | 97 |
|   |   | 5.2.2 | Active Targeting and Tumour Selectivity | 97 |
|   |   | 5.2.3 | Overcoming Tumour Hypoxia | 97 |
|   |   | 5.2.4 | Deep-Tumour PDT: Up Conversion and X-ray Activation | 98 |
|   |   | 5.2.5 | Stimuli-Responsive and Combinatorial Systems | 99 |
|   |   | 5.2.6 | Clinical Translation and Challenges | 100 |
|   | 5.3 | | Nanocrystal Surface Engineering for Enhanced Photothermal and Photodynamic Efficiency | 100 |
|   | 5.4 | | Common Features and Synergistic Potential of Photothermal and Photodynamic Therapy | 101 |
|   | 5.5 | | Integration of PTT and PDT with Other Modalities: Synergistic Strategies for Advanced Cancer Therapy | 101 |
|   |   | 5.5.1 | Chemotherapy: Enhancing Drug Delivery and Overcoming Resistance | 103 |
|   |   | 5.5.2 | Radiotherapy: Oxygenation and Radio Sensitization | 103 |
|   |   | 5.5.3 | Gene Therapy and Immunotherapy: Reprogramming the Tumour Microenvironment | 104 |
|   | 5.6 | | Future Directions and Challenges | 104 |
|   | References | | | 106 |
| 6 | **Imaging, Diagnostics, and Theranostics Applications of Nanocrystals** | | | **113** |
|   | 6.1 | | Introduction | 113 |
|   | 6.2 | | NCs in the Detection of Cancer Biomarkers | 114 |
|   | 6.3 | | NCs' Application in Imaging and Diagnosis of Cancer | 117 |
|   |   | 6.3.1 | NCs in MRI | 118 |
|   |   | 6.3.2 | NCs in CT | 119 |
|   |   | 6.3.3 | NCs in Fluorescent Imaging | 123 |
|   |   | 6.3.4 | NCs in Multimodal Imaging of Cancer | 124 |
|   | 6.4 | | NCs in the Cancer Theranostics | 125 |
|   | 6.5 | | Conclusion | 130 |
|   | References | | | 130 |
| 7 | **Toxicity, Clinical Studies of Nanocrystals, Conclusion and Future Scope** | | | **139** |
|   | 7.1 | | Toxicity of Nanocrystals | 139 |
|   |   | 7.1.1 | Hydrophilic Nanocrystals | 140 |
|   |   | 7.1.2 | Organic Nanocrystals | 141 |
|   |   | 7.1.3 | Lipid-Based Nanoparticles | 141 |
|   |   | 7.1.4 | Bioinspired Nanocrystals | 141 |

|   |   |   |
|---|---|---|
| | 7.1.5 Metal–Organic Framework | 143 |
| | 7.1.6 Quantum Dots (QD) | 143 |
| | 7.1.7 Carbon Dots (CD) and Carbon-Based Nanocrystals | 145 |
| | 7.1.8 Inorganic Nanocrystals | 145 |
| 7.2 | Clinical Studies of Nanocrystals | 147 |
| 7.3 | Conclusion | 154 |
| 7.4 | Future Scope | 156 |
| References | | 157 |

# Introduction

Cancer continues to be a central cause of mortality globally. Cancer comprehends over 200 different diseases, each with distinct molecular backgrounds, genetic mutations, and phenotypic characteristics [1–3]. It remains one of the foremost health challenges of the twenty-first century, accounting for nearly 10 million deaths globally each year [4, 5]. Despite significant strides in early detection, surgical techniques, radiation, and systemic therapies, cancer continues to escape cure in many cases due to its intrinsic biological complexity, malleability, and heterogeneity [1, 6–8]. One of the fundamental limitations of current treatment modalities is their failure to precisely differentiate between cancerous and healthy cells, resulting in off-target toxicity, treatment failure, and the development of resistance mechanisms [8–10].

Upon closer examination of the problems with different treatment modalities, such as chemotherapy, which is frequently assigned as the first-line systemic treatment for several cancers, reveals that several pharmacological and biological flaws specifically limit its effectiveness [11–13]. These include poor bioavailability due to rapid clearance or degradation, as well as nonspecific biodistribution, which can result in drug accumulation in healthy tissues [13, 14]. Lack of selectivity results in cytotoxic effects that are subjective, affecting both cancerous and normal cells [9, 15, 16]. These inherent limitations not only reduce the therapeutic efficacy of chemotherapeutic agents but also contribute to severe systemic toxicity, treatment resistance, and reduced quality of life for patients [16–18]. Similarly. However, radiation therapy is premeditated to target tumor sites precisely, and it often results in collateral damage to immediate healthy tissues due to the limited ability to confine ionizing radiation exclusively to cancer cells [19, 20]. This unintended exposure can damage normal tissue function, lead to inflammation and fibrosis, and, in some cases, induce genetic mutations that increase the long-term risk of developing secondary malignancies [21–24].

Notwithstanding advancements in imaging and delivery techniques, these off-target effects remain a significant limitation of radiation-based cancer treatment [25, 26]. Equally, immunotherapies and targeted therapies have revolutionized cancer treatment by introducing precision-based methods that exploit specific molecular or immunological features of tumors [27–29]. However, their clinical efficiency is often controlled by several challenges [30–32]. Tumor cells can develop mechanisms of immune evasion, such as creating an immunosuppressive microenvironment and downregulating antigen presentation, which weakens the efficacy of immune-based treatments [33–35]. Additionally, antigenic heterogeneity, both within a single tumor and across patients, obscures the design of targeted agents that are universally effective [36, 37].

These therapies also present significant financial challenges, which limit accessibility and hinder their widespread clinical adoption [38, 39]. Together, these factors present significant hurdles to the long-term success and scalability of these otherwise promising modalities. Moreover, a significant and growing challenge is the development of multidrug resistance (MDR), where cancer cells acquire or inherit personalities that reduce their sensitivity to a broad range of therapeutics, thereby severely compromising treatment efficacy [40–42]. In summary, these issues highlight the pressing need for innovative strategies that can improve therapeutic outcomes while minimizing adverse side effects [8, 43, 44].

Such obstacles not only diminish the quality of life for patients but also highlight the essential and urgent need for innovative therapeutic strategies [45, 46]. These new approaches must focus on enhancing precision in targeting cancer cells while sparing healthy ones, improving overall therapeutic outcomes, and significantly minimizing adverse reactions to ensure a better quality of life for those affected by this pervasive disease [47]. In response to these limitations, the integration of nanotechnology into oncology has reformed the landscape of cancer therapy and diagnostics, giving rise to the field of cancer theranostics [48–50]. This prototype combines diagnostic and therapeutic functions into a single nanoplatform [51]. The application of nanotechnology in cancer medicine has garnered unprecedented attention over the last two decades [52, 53]. The convergence of nanoscience, molecular biology, and oncology has given rise to a new field called cancer theranostics [50]. This integrated approach combines therapeutic and diagnostic functionalities within a single nanoscale platform [54]. Among the various nanostructures being explored, including liposomes, micelles, dendrimers, and polymeric nanoparticles, nanocrystals have emerged as a promising class of materials [55, 56] due to their unique physicochemical qualities, including high surface area-to-volume ratios, tunable size, and shape, the ability to encapsulate or conjugate a wide range of therapeutic and imaging agents and the capacity for multifunctionalization [55, 57]. These attributes enable nanocrystals to serve as efficient drug delivery vehicles, enhance the precision of targeted therapies, and facilitate real-time monitoring of treatment response through advanced imaging modalities [58, 59].

## 1.1 What Are Nanocrystals?

Nanocrystals are crystalline structures comprised of a few hundred to a few thousand atoms, typically measuring less than 100 nm in diameter [60]. Unlike amorphous nanoparticles, nanocrystals exhibit long-range atomic order, well-defined lattice structures, and highly tunable morphologies, such as rods, spheres, sheets, and cubes [61–63]. These characteristics reveal them with astonishing optical, electrical, magnetic, and catalytic properties that are not present in their bulk counterparts [56, 63]. These can be synthesized from a wide variety of organic, inorganic, or hybrid materials [64, 65]. Their defining characteristics render them uniquely suited for biomedical applications [66]. These include the encapsulation or conjugation of therapeutic agents, active targeting ligands, and imaging probes, allowing nanocrystals to serve as multifunctional platforms that enhance drug solubility, stability, and biodistribution while reducing off-target effects [57, 67–69]. Depending on their composition, nanocrystals may be organic, such as crystalline drug molecules or conjugated polymers, inorganic, like metal, metal oxide, or semiconductor crystals, or hybrid systems that incorporate both organic and inorganic components for synergistic functionality [69, 70]. Their large surface area-to-volume ratio enables high drug loading capacity, and their surfaces can be functionalized with targeting ligands, polymers, or stimuli-responsive moieties to enhance biocompatibility, prolong circulation time, and increase specificity [71, 72]. Their versatility extends to applications such as targeted drug delivery, immunomodulation, photothermal and photodynamic therapies, and multimodal imaging, making them integral to the next generation of personalized cancer care [73, 74]. Furthermore, ongoing research into the biophysical characterization, toxicity profiles, and clinical translation of nanocrystals continues to expand their potential for safe and effective integration into routine oncology practice [58].

A defining feature of nanocrystals in theranostics is their dual functionality in diagnostics and therapy [55]. Nanocrystals can be labeled with or inherently possess imaging capabilities, enabling real-time tracking of biodistribution, accumulation, and therapeutic response using imaging modalities such as MRI, PET, fluorescence, or photoacoustic imaging [57, 75]. This capacity for image-guided therapy represents a significant advancement in personalized medicine, as clinicians can monitor treatment efficacy and adjust regimens accordingly [76, 77].

The versatility of nanocrystals encompasses a broad spectrum of material platforms, each offering distinct physicochemical and functional advantages that can be strategically leveraged for biomedical applications:

## 1.1.1 Organic Nanocrystals

Organic nanocrystals, including liposomes, dendrimers, and polymeric nanoparticles, are praised for their intrinsic biocompatibility, biodegradability, and tunable surface chemistry [78, 79]. These systems offer a high degree of enterprise flexibility, enabling the incorporation of targeting ligands, stealth polymers (e.g., PEG), or responsive moieties to facilitate site-specific delivery, prolonged circulation, and controlled drug release [60, 80].

## 1.1.2 Inorganic Nanocrystals

Inorganic nanocrystals, such as iron oxide, gold nanoparticles, silica, and quantum dots, exhibit remarkable structural stability and unique physicochemical attributes, including surface plasmon resonance, magnetic susceptibility, and fluorescence. These properties make them exceptionally well-suited for applications in molecular imaging (MRI, CT, optical), photothermal and photodynamic therapies, as well as biosensing [81].

## 1.1.3 Hybrid Nanocrystals

Hybrid nanocrystals represent a convergent class of nanomaterials that synergistically combine the biological compatibility of organic components with the functional versatility of inorganic cores [82, 83]. This hybridization enables integrated theranostic capabilities, such as simultaneous imaging, real-time drug tracking, and stimuli-triggered therapeutic payload release, positioning them at the forefront of personalized nanomedicine [84, 85].

## 1.2 Functional Properties of Nanocrystals

Nanocrystals possess a diverse range of functional properties that arise from their material composition, dimensionality, and surface chemistry [60, 86]. These properties enable their use in advanced biomedical applications, including targeted drug delivery, diagnostic imaging, and therapeutic intervention [69]. Their functionalities are typically categorized based on whether the nanocrystals are organic or inorganic in nature.

## 1.2.1 Organic Nanocrystals

Organic nanocrystals, comprising lipid-based, polymeric, and dendrimeric systems, exhibit several functional characteristics that are critical for therapeutic and diagnostic versatility [87, 88]. Many organic nanocrystals, such as liposomes and polymeric micelles, display amphiphilic architectures, allowing them to encapsulate both hydrophilic and hydrophobic drugs simultaneously [89]. This dual-loading capability enhances combination therapy strategies and pharmacokinetic control. Furthermore, their surfaces can be readily modified with targeting ligands, like folic acid, hyaluronic acid, or antibodies, to achieve receptor-mediated delivery to specific cell types or tumor microenvironments [90]. Certain organic nanocrystals, especially those composed of aromatic or π-conjugated systems, for example, polydopamine, porphyrins, diketopyrrolopyrrole derivatives, exhibit nonlinear optical behaviors such as second harmonic generation (SHG) and two-photon absorption. These photonic traits are valuable for advanced bioimaging techniques and photodynamic therapy applications, enabling deeper tissue penetration and real-time visualization [91].

### 1.2.2 Inorganic Nanocrystals

Inorganic nanocrystals, which include metallic, magnetic, and semiconductor-based materials, are prized for their robust physical properties and tunable size-dependent functionalities [92]. At the nanoscale, inorganic crystals such as gold nanoparticles, iron oxide, quantum dots, and upconversion nanoparticles exhibit size- and shape-dependent optical, electronic, and magnetic behaviors [93]. For example, gold nanoparticles can be tuned to absorb near-infrared light, enabling their use in photothermal therapy by converting light energy into localized heat for the ablation of tumors [94]. Similarly, iron oxide nanoparticles possess superparamagnetic properties suitable for magnetic resonance imaging (MRI) contrast enhancement and magnetically guided drug delivery [95].

High atomic number (Z) inorganic nanocrystals, particularly those based on gold, hafnium oxide, and bismuth sulfide, can amplify the effects of ionizing radiation by enhancing local radiation dose deposition [96]. This phenomenon, known as radiosensitization, improves the therapeutic index of radiotherapy, particularly in hypoxic or radioresistant tumors [97]. Many inorganic nanocrystals also exhibit enzyme-mimetic (nanozyme) activity or redox properties that can modulate the tumor microenvironment. For example, cerium oxide nanoparticles can scavenge reactive oxygen species (ROS), while manganese oxide can generate oxygen in situ, helping overcome hypoxia-induced therapy resistance [98].

### 1.2.3 Hybrid Nanocrystals

Similarly, Hybrid nanocrystals that integrate both organic and inorganic domains further extend these functional benefits by enabling multimodal imaging, synergistic drug action, and stimuli-responsive release mechanisms, blending biological compatibility with physicochemical precision [99].

## 1.3 Biocompatibility and Toxicity

The biocompatibility and potential toxicity of nanocrystals are critical factors influencing their clinical translation, especially for applications involving systemic administration or long-term exposure [100]. These properties are highly dependent on the material composition, surface chemistry, size, and degradation profile of the nanocrystals [101].

### 1.3.1 Organic Nanocrystals

Organic nanocrystals, such as those composed of lipids, polymers, or dendrimers, are generally regarded as highly biocompatible due to their chemical similarity to naturally occurring biomolecules [102]. These systems tend to degrade into non-toxic byproducts that are readily metabolized or excreted, making them particularly suitable for systemic drug delivery and long-term therapeutic use [103]. Surface modification strategies, such as PEGylation (attachment of polyethylene glycol chains), significantly enhance the stealth characteristics of organic nanocarriers by reducing opsonization and clearance by the mononuclear phagocyte system (MPS) [104]. For instance, PEGylated liposomes, such as those used in FDA-approved formulations (e.g., Doxil), exhibit prolonged circulation times and reduced immune recognition [105]. Many organic carriers are constructed from materials such as PLGA, chitosan, or phospholipids, which undergo enzymatic or hydrolytic degradation. This biodegradability reduces the risk of long-term accumulation and supports their use in repeat dosing regimens [106].

### 1.3.2 Inorganic Nanocrystals

In contrast, inorganic nanocrystals pose more complex challenges regarding biocompatibility and toxicity, primarily due to their elemental composition, poor biodegradability, and the potential for bioaccumulation [107]. Certain inorganic materials, such as quantum dots containing cadmium or lead, raise concerns due to the release of heavy metals under physiological conditions [108]. These ions can interfere with cellular processes, induce oxidative stress and exhibit genotoxic effects. Inorganic nanocrystals often resist enzymatic breakdown, leading to prolonged retention in organs such as the liver, spleen, and lungs [109]. Chronic exposure or repeated administration may result in cumulative toxicity, particularly for non-degradable systems [110]. To enhance safety profiles, surface engineering approaches are employed, including encapsulation with biocompatible coatings like silica, PEG, or zwitterionic polymers [111]. These layers help minimize direct contact between toxic cores and biological systems, improve dispersibility, and reduce immune activation [112]. Overall, while organic nanocrystals offer a favorable safety profile conducive to clinical translation, inorganic systems require careful design and surface modification to balance their enhanced functionalities with acceptable biocompatibility [102, 113]. Ongoing research aims to optimize hybrid systems that retain the advantages of both platforms while minimizing their respective risks [114].

## 1.4 Synthesis and Applications of Nanocrystals

The synthesis methods and functional applications of nanocrystals are deeply influenced by their material class, organic or inorganic. While both types offer unique advantages, their production techniques, stability, and biomedical applications differ significantly, shaping their suitability for various therapeutic and diagnostic roles [115].

### 1.4.1 Synthesis of Organic Nanocrystals

Organic nanocrystals are typically synthesized using bottom-up self-assembly techniques, where amphiphilic molecules such as phospholipids, polymers, or dendrimers spontaneously organize into nanoscale structures in aqueous environments [115, 116]. Hydrophobic interactions, electrostatic forces, or hydrogen bonding often drive this process. Although the self-assembly method enables the creation of biocompatible, soft-matter systems, it requires precise control over solvent conditions, pH, and ionic strength to ensure uniformity and prevent unwanted aggregation or precipitation [102]. Importantly, organic nanomaterials can be designed to be recyclable or biodegradable, supporting sustainable and safe biomedical use [117]. Organic nanocrystals are extensively used in drug delivery systems, with liposomes, polymeric micelles, and dendrimer-based carriers leading the way. These nanocarriers can capture a wide range of therapeutic agents, protect them from premature degradation, and enable controlled or stimuli-responsive release [70, 114]. In addition to pharmaceutical delivery, organic nanocrystals are also employed in light-harvesting systems for bioimaging or photodynamic therapy due to their tunable optical properties. Moreover, their biodegradability and mechanical versatility make them suitable for temporary biomedical implants, tissue scaffolds, and wound dressings that gradually degrade without eliciting adverse immune responses [118].

### 1.4.2 Synthesis of Inorganic Nanocrystals

Inorganic nanocrystals are typically synthesized via colloidal chemical methods, which allow for highly controlled nucleation and growth processes [119, 120]. Techniques such as thermal decomposition, sol–gel synthesis, and hydrothermal methods enable precise tuning of particle size, morphology (e.g., spheres, rods, stars), and surface chemistry

[121]. For instance, the synthesis of gold nanorods can be finely tuned to manipulate their longitudinal plasmon resonance, making them ideal for plasmonic imaging and photothermal therapy [122]. Surface functionalization strategies further enhance their targeting, dispersion, and stability in biological environments [123]. Inorganic nanocrystals exhibit diverse and often multifunctional applications in biomedicine due to their distinctive optical, magnetic, and catalytic properties [92]. Quantum dots, for example, are used in biosensing and fluorescence-based imaging owing to their high brightness and photostability [124]. Titanium dioxide ($TiO_2$) nanoparticles are widely employed in photodynamic therapy, where light-activated ROS production leads to localized tumor cell destruction [125]. Iron oxide nanoparticles possess magnetic properties suitable for magnetic resonance imaging (MRI), magnetic targeting, and thermal ablation (hyperthermia) therapy, where they generate heat under alternating magnetic fields to kill cancer cells [126]. In summary, the synthesis routes for organic and inorganic nanocrystals differ fundamentally in their mechanisms and control parameters, which in turn influence their functional applications. Organic systems excel in biocompatible therapeutic delivery and implantable devices, while inorganic platforms offer precision diagnostics and energy-driven therapies together, forming a powerful toolkit for modern nanomedicine.

## 1.5 Therapeutic Applications and Mechanisms

### 1.5.1 Enhanced Drug Delivery and Tumor Targeting

Nanocrystals preferentially accumulate in tumor tissues via the enhanced permeability and retention (EPR) effect, exploiting leaky vasculature and impaired lymphatic drainage to increase local drug concentrations and reduce systemic exposure [127]. Functionalization with ligands (e.g., hyaluronic acid) enables nanocrystals to bind selectively to overexpressed receptors (e.g., CD44), thereby enhancing uptake by cancer cells [128]. For instance, anthocyanin-doxorubicin nanocrystals effectively target CD44+ cancer cells, promoting apoptosis while sparing healthy tissues [129].

### 1.5.2 Controlled Drug Release

pH-sensitive nanocrystals release their payload in acidic tumor microenvironments, ensuring site-specific action [130]. For example, iron oxide nanozymes paired with ascorbic acid demonstrate potent cytotoxicity only upon cellular internalization [131].

## 1.5 Therapeutic Applications and Mechanisms

### 1.5.3 Overcoming Multidrug Resistance

Encapsulation shields drugs from recognition by efflux transporters like P-glycoprotein [132]. Anthocyanin-loaded nanocarriers, for example, have been shown to mitigate cisplatin resistance in ovarian cancer models [133]. Co-loaded formulations (e.g., camptothecin and all-trans retinoic acid) exhibit synergistic effects, suppressing cancer stem cell populations and reducing the likelihood of recurrence [134].

### 1.5.4 Radiotherapy Enhancement

Inorganic nanocrystals with high atomic numbers (e.g., gold) enhance radiotherapy by increasing ionization and secondary electron generation, thereby reducing the required radiation dose and limiting toxicity [135].

### 1.5.5 Immunomodulation and Combination Therapies

Magnetic nanocrystals embedded in macrophages can be externally directed to tumor sites, amplifying localized treatment effects, such as ascorbic acid-mediated cytotoxicity. These formulations enhance drug solubility and bioavailability while minimizing adverse reactions. For example, albumin-bound paclitaxel allows for higher tolerated doses with fewer side effects.

### 1.5.6 Reduced Systemic Toxicity

Nanocrystals reduce premature degradation and prevent widespread drug diffusion, sparing healthy cells. PEGylated liposomal doxorubicin, for example, exhibits reduced cardiotoxicity compared to its free-form counterpart [136]. Nanocrystals improve solubility, prolong circulation, and enable targeted accumulation in tumors [137].

Nanocrystals modulate immune responses, deliver cytokines, or target immune cells to tumors. Integration with imaging modalities enables the visualization of tumors and the biodistribution of nanocrystals [138]. Co-delivery of multiple agents in a single nanocrystal platform addresses tumor heterogeneity [139]. By bringing together the latest advances and expert perspectives, this volume aims to serve as an important resource for investigators, clinicians, and students interested in connecting the power of nanocrystals for transformative progress in cancer theranostics [140]. By integrating these mechanisms, nanocrystals address critical limitations of conventional therapies, offering a versatile platform for personalized and multimodal cancer treatment [57].

## 1.6 Translational Challenges and Clinical Outlook

Despite the scientific promise, translating nanocrystals from laboratory bench to clinical bedside is not without challenges. Key issues include the scalability and reproducibility of nanocrystal synthesis under Good Manufacturing Practices (GMP). Comprehensive safety profiling, including biodistribution, immunogenicity, long-term toxicity, and clearance mechanisms. Regulatory approval hurdles, as multifunctional theranostic agents do not fit neatly into traditional drug or device categories. Inter-patient variability in tumor vascularity and EPR effect may influence targeting efficiency. Cost-effectiveness and accessibility of complex nanocrystal formulations in global healthcare settings. Nonetheless, several nanocrystal-based formulations are already in clinical trials, and a few, such as albumin-bound paclitaxel (Abraxane®), have received regulatory approval, validating the clinical feasibility of such platforms. These capabilities collectively enable nanocrystals to function as theranostic agent platforms that not only deliver therapeutic payloads but also facilitate real-time tracking of drug delivery, monitoring of treatment efficacy, and early disease diagnosis, all while minimizing systemic toxicity.

## 1.7 Scope of This Book

This book, Nanocrystals in Cancer Theranostics, aims to provide a comprehensive and multidisciplinary overview of the design, development, and application of nanocrystals for cancer diagnosis and treatment. It begins by initiating the underlying principles of nanocrystal synthesis and characterization, then delves into their use in targeted drug delivery, imaging, radiosensitization, immunotherapy, and combination therapies. Special attention is given to emerging trends, including stimuli-responsive nanocrystals, modulation of the tumor microenvironment, and personalized nanomedicine. Each chapter integrates current research findings with practical considerations for clinical translation, making this volume a valuable resource for academic researchers, pharmaceutical scientists, oncologists, biomedical engineers, and students seeking to advance their understanding of nanotechnology's role in combating cancer.

By bridging the gap between nanoscience and clinical oncology, this book seeks to inspire new ideas, adoptive collaboration, and fast-track the development of transformative treatments that can advance survival and quality of life for cancer patients worldwide.

## 1.8 Structure of This Book

This book, Nanocrystals in Cancer Theranostics, seeks to provide an authoritative and interdisciplinary exploration of this rapidly advancing field. Structured to appeal to both novices and experts, the text is organized into the following sections:

- **Fundamental Principles**: An overview of nanocrystal types, synthesis methods, physicochemical characterization, and functionalization strategies.
- **Therapeutic Applications**: In-depth discussions on nanocrystal-mediated chemotherapy, photothermal therapy, immunotherapy, and radiosensitization.
- **Diagnostic and Imaging Techniques**: Integration of nanocrystals into modalities like MRI, CT, fluorescence, and multimodal imaging systems.
- **Translational and Clinical Perspectives**: Case studies of preclinical and clinical candidates, safety assessment, regulatory pathways, and future challenges.

By combining fundamental science with translational insight, this volume aims to serve as a comprehensive reference for materials scientists, pharmaceutical researchers, clinicians, bioengineers, and graduate students. It also aspires to bridge the gap between discovery and application, ultimately contributing to the design of safer, more effective, and personalized cancer therapies. As the field of nanomedicine evolves, nanocrystals are poised to become central components of the oncology toolbox, transforming the way we diagnose, monitor, and treat cancer. This book stands as both a reflection of past achievements and a blueprint for the future—where precision, integration, and innovation redefine the fight against cancer.

## 1.9 Conclusion

Nanocrystals offer a robust and adaptable platform for addressing some of the most persistent challenges in oncology. From improving drug solubility and selectivity to enabling real-time imaging and overcoming resistance, these materials have established themselves as a cornerstone of next-generation cancer theranostics. As research continues to refine their design and safety profiles, nanocrystal-based technologies are poised for broader clinical translation, paving the way for more effective, personalized, and less toxic cancer therapies. This book serves as both a foundational resource and a forward-looking guide, uniting fundamental principles with translational strategies to inspire innovation and foster collaboration across the domains of nanotechnology, oncology, and personalized medicine.

## References

1. HASAN, D. S. (2024). *INTRODUCTION TO CANCER BIOLOGY AND GENETICS: Cancer Genetics Unlocked*: Notion Press.
2. Tiwari, L., & Kujan, O. (2025). Molecular Basis of Cancer. *Pathological Basis of Oral and Maxillofacial Diseases*, 415–428.

3. Wang, L., Gu, M., Zhang, X., Kong, T., Liao, J., Zhang, D., et al. (2025). Recent Advances in Nanoenzymes Based Therapies for Glioblastoma: Overcoming Barriers and Enhancing Targeted Treatment. *Advanced Science*, 2413367.
4. Ng, M., Gakidou, E., Lo, J., Abate, Y. H., Abbafati, C., Abbas, N., et al. (2025). Global, regional, and national prevalence of adult overweight and obesity, 1990–2021, with forecasts to 2050: a forecasting study for the Global Burden of Disease Study 2021. *The Lancet, 405*(10481), 813–838.
5. Sobti, R. C., Gosipatala, S. B., Sharma, M., Reddy, P., Khalko, R. K., Kaur, T., et al. (2023). Types of Cancers, Epidemiology, and Molecular Insights. In *Handbook of Oncobiology: From Basic to Clinical Sciences* (pp. 1–36): Springer.
6. Du, W., & Elemento, O. (2015). Cancer systems biology: embracing complexity to develop better anticancer therapeutic strategies. *Oncogene, 34*(25), 3215–3225.
7. Fuloria, N. K., Malviya, R., Verma, S., & Balusamy, B. (2023). *Big Data in Oncology: Impact, Challenges, and Risk Assessment*: CRC Press.
8. Garg, P., Malhotra, J., Kulkarni, P., Horne, D., Salgia, R., & Singhal, S. S. (2024). Emerging therapeutic strategies to overcome drug resistance in cancer cells. *Cancers, 16*(13), 2478.
9. Liu, B., Zhou, H., Tan, L., Siu, K. T. H., & Guan, X.-Y. (2024). Exploring treatment options in cancer: tumor treatment strategies. *Signal transduction and targeted therapy, 9*(1), 175.
10. Kaur, R., Bhardwaj, A., & Gupta, S. (2023). Cancer treatment therapies: traditional to modern approaches to combat cancers. *Molecular biology reports, 50*(11), 9663–9676.
11. Anand, U., Dey, A., Chandel, A. K. S., Sanyal, R., Mishra, A., Pandey, D. K., et al. (2023). Cancer chemotherapy and beyond: Current status, drug candidates, associated risks and progress in targeted therapeutics. *Genes & diseases, 10*(4), 1367–1401.
12. Kuderer, N. M., Desai, A., Lustberg, M. B., & Lyman, G. H. (2022). Mitigating acute chemotherapy-associated adverse events in patients with cancer. *Nature Reviews Clinical Oncology, 19*(11), 681–697.
13. Han, H., Chen, B.-T., Liu, Y., Wang, Y., Xing, L., Wang, H., et al. (2024). Engineered stem cell-based strategy: A new paradigm of next-generation stem cell product in regenerative medicine. *Journal of Controlled Release, 365*, 981–1003.
14. Cavalcanti, I. D. L., & Soares, J. C. S. (2021). *Advances in Cancer Treatment: From Systemic Chemotherapy to Targeted Therapy*: Springer Nature.
15. Bracci, L., Schiavoni, G., Sistigu, A., & Belardelli, F. (2014). Immune-based mechanisms of cytotoxic chemotherapy: implications for the design of novel and rationale-based combined treatments against cancer. *Cell Death & Differentiation, 21*(1), 15–25.
16. Sharma, M., Bakshi, A. K., Mittapelly, N., Gautam, S., Marwaha, D., Rai, N., et al. (2022). Recent updates on innovative approaches to overcome drug resistance for better outcomes in cancer. *Journal of Controlled Release, 346*, 43–70.
17. Eslami, M., Memarsadeghi, O., Davarpanah, A., Arti, A., Nayernia, K., & Behnam, B. (2024). Overcoming chemotherapy resistance in metastatic cancer: a comprehensive review. *Biomedicines, 12*(1), 183.
18. Ingole, S., Vasdev, N., Tekade, M., Gupta, T., Pawar, B., Mhatre, M., et al. (2024). Toxic effects of cancer therapies. In *Public Health and Toxicology Issues Drug Research, Volume 2* (pp. 353–379): Elsevier.
19. Dhakad, G. G., Patil, G. D., Nikum, A. C., & Shirsat, S. P. (2022). Review on radiation therapy on cancer. *Research Journal of Pharmacology and Pharmacodynamics, 14*(1), 4–12.
20. Biswal, B. M., Nee, L. F., & Appalanaido, G. K. (2025). Early and Late Toxicities of Radiotherapy. In *Radiation Oncology–Principles, Precepts and Practice: Volume I–Technical Aspects* (pp. 383–407): Springer.

21. Wang, K., & Tepper, J. E. (2021). Radiation therapy-associated toxicity: Etiology, management, and prevention. *CA: a cancer journal for clinicians, 71*(5), 437–454.
22. Yu, Z., Xu, C., Song, B., Zhang, S., Chen, C., Li, C., et al. (2023). Tissue fibrosis induced by radiotherapy: current understanding of the molecular mechanisms, diagnosis and therapeutic advances. *Journal of translational medicine, 21*(1), 708.
23. Wang, H., Zou, W., & Cao, Y. (2025). Radiation-induced cellular senescence and adaptive response: mechanistic interplay and implications. *Radiation Medicine and Protection*.
24. Sárközy, M., Varga, Z., Gáspár, R., Szűcs, G., Kovács, M. G., Kovács, Z. Z., et al. (2021). Pathomechanisms and therapeutic opportunities in radiation-induced heart disease: from bench to bedside. *Clinical Research in Cardiology, 110*(4), 507–531.
25. Pazzaglia, S., Eidemüller, M., Lumniczky, K., Mancuso, M., Ramadan, R., Stolarczyk, L., et al. (2022). Out-of-field effects: lessons learned from partial body exposure. *Radiation and Environmental Biophysics, 61*(4), 485–504.
26. Hull, R., Mbodi, L., Hadebe, B., Sartor, O., & Dlamini, Z. (2024). Radiopharmaceuticals and Radiotherapy: Advances in Radiation-Based Therapies. In *Transforming Prostate Cancer Care: Advancing Cancer Treatment with Insights from Africa* (pp. 149–169): Springer.
27. Mohite, P., Yadav, V., Pandhare, R., Maitra, S., Saleh, F. M., Saleem, R. M., et al. (2024). Revolutionizing cancer treatment: unleashing the power of viral vaccines, monoclonal antibodies, and proteolysis-targeting chimeras in the new era of immunotherapy. *ACS omega, 9*(7), 7277–7295.
28. Kiani, M. N., Khaliq, H., Abubakar, M., Rafique, M., Jalilov, F., Ashraf, G. A., et al. (2025). Advancing the potential of nanoparticles for cancer detection and precision therapeutics. *Medical Oncology, 42*(7), 1–32.
29. Lin, Y., Lin, P., Xu, R., Chen, X., Lu, Y., Zheng, J., et al. (2025). Nanovaccines empowering CD8+ T cells: a precision strategy to enhance cancer immunotherapy. *Theranostics, 15*(7), 3098.
30. Yang, R., Li, Y., Wang, H., Qin, T., Yin, X., & Ma, X. (2022). Therapeutic progress and challenges for triple negative breast cancer: targeted therapy and immunotherapy. *Molecular biomedicine, 3*(1), 8.
31. Taefehshokr, S., Parhizkar, A., Hayati, S., Mousapour, M., Mahmoudpour, A., Eleid, L., et al. (2022). Cancer immunotherapy: Challenges and limitations. *Pathology-Research and Practice, 229*, 153723.
32. Aldea, M., Andre, F., Marabelle, A., Dogan, S., Barlesi, F., & Soria, J.-C. (2021). Overcoming resistance to tumor-targeted and immune-targeted therapies. *Cancer Discovery, 11*(4), 874–899.
33. Imani, S., Farghadani, R., Roozitalab, G., Maghsoudloo, M., Emadi, M., Moradi, A., et al. (2025). Reprogramming the breast tumor immune microenvironment: cold-to-hot transition for enhanced immunotherapy. *J Exp Clin Cancer Res, 44*(1), 131, https://doi.org/10.1186/s13046-025-03394-8.
34. Gu, C., Sha, G., Zeng, B., Cao, H., Cao, Y., & Tang, D. (2025). Therapeutic potential of fecal microbiota transplantation in colorectal cancer based on gut microbiota regulation: from pathogenesis to efficacy. *Therap Adv Gastroenterol, 18*, 17562848251327167, https://doi.org/10.1177/17562848251327167.
35. Lin, X., Kang, K., Chen, P., Zeng, Z., Li, G., Xiong, W., et al. (2024). Regulatory mechanisms of PD-1/PD-L1 in cancers. *Mol Cancer, 23*(1), 108, https://doi.org/10.1186/s12943-024-02023-w.
36. Zhang, X., Xie, J., Yang, Z., Yu, C. K. W., Hu, Y., & Qin, J. (2025). Tumour heterogeneity and personalized treatment screening based on single-cell transcriptomics. *Computational and Structural Biotechnology Journal, 27*, 307–320, https://doi.org/10.1016/j.csbj.2024.12.020

37. Sun, X.-x., & Yu, Q. (2015). Intra-tumor heterogeneity of cancer cells and its implications for cancer treatment. *Acta Pharmacologica Sinica, 36*(10), 1219–1227, https://doi.org/10.1038/aps.2015.92.
38. Htwe, O., Yuliawiratman, B. S., Tannor, A. Y., Nor Asikin, M. Z., Soh, E., W, D. E. G., et al. (2024). Barriers and facilitators for increased accessibility to quality rehabilitation services in low- and middle- income countries: a systematic review. *Eur J Phys Rehabil Med, 60*(3), 514–522, https://doi.org/10.23736/s1973-9087.24.08154-1.
39. Marchal, I. (2025). Making cell therapy accessible: challenges and opportunities. *Nature Biotechnology, 43*(4), 482–486, https://doi.org/10.1038/s41587-025-02625-9.
40. Mengistu, B. A., Tsegaw, T., Demessie, Y., Getnet, K., Bitew, A. B., Kinde, M. Z., et al. (2024). Comprehensive review of drug resistance in mammalian cancer stem cells: implications for cancer therapy. *Cancer Cell International, 24*(1), 406, https://doi.org/10.1186/s12935-024-03558-0.
41. Emran, T. B., Shahriar, A., Mahmud, A. R., Rahman, T., Abir, M. H., Siddiquee, M. F., et al. (2022). Multidrug Resistance in Cancer: Understanding Molecular Mechanisms, Immunoprevention and Therapeutic Approaches. *Front Oncol, 12*, 891652, https://doi.org/10.3389/fonc.2022.891652.
42. Duan, C., Yu, M., Xu, J., Li, B.-Y., Zhao, Y., & Kankala, R. K. (2023). Overcoming Cancer Multi-drug Resistance (MDR): Reasons, mechanisms, nanotherapeutic solutions, and challenges. *Biomedicine & Pharmacotherapy, 162*, 114643.
43. Ezike, T. C., Okpala, U. S., Onoja, U. L., Nwike, C. P., Ezeako, E. C., Okpara, O. J., et al. (2023). Advances in drug delivery systems, challenges and future directions. *Heliyon, 9*(6), e17488, https://doi.org/10.1016/j.heliyon.2023.e17488.
44. Connor, L., Dean, J., McNett, M., Tydings, D. M., Shrout, A., Gorsuch, P. F., et al. (2023). Evidence-based practice improves patient outcomes and healthcare system return on investment: Findings from a scoping review. *Worldviews Evid Based Nurs, 20*(1), 6–15, https://doi.org/10.1111/wvn.12621.
45. Sharma, D., & Cotton, M. (2023). Overcoming the barriers between resource constraints and healthcare quality. *Tropical Doctor, 53*(3), 341–343, https://doi.org/10.1177/00494755231183784.
46. Kumah, A. (2025). Poor quality care in healthcare settings: an overlooked epidemic. [Review]. *Frontiers in Public Health, Volume 13 - 2025*, https://doi.org/10.3389/fpubh.2025.1504172.
47. Sabit, H., Pawlik, T. M., Radwan, F., Abdel-Hakeem, M., Abdel-Ghany, S., Wadan, A.-H. S., et al. (2025). Precision nanomedicine: navigating the tumor microenvironment for enhanced cancer immunotherapy and targeted drug delivery. *Molecular Cancer, 24*(1), 160, https://doi.org/10.1186/s12943-025-02357-z.
48. Rehan, F., Zhang, M., Fang, J., & Greish, K. (2024). Therapeutic applications of nanomedicine: recent developments and future perspectives. *Molecules, 29*(9), 2073.
49. Gavas, S., Quazi, S., & Karpiński, T. M. (2021). Nanoparticles for Cancer Therapy: Current Progress and Challenges. *Nanoscale Res Lett, 16*(1), 173, https://doi.org/10.1186/s11671-021-03628-6.
50. Teng, L., Bi, Y., Xing, X., & Yao, G. (2025). Nano-oncology revisited: Insights on precise therapeutic advances and challenges in tumor. *Fundamental Research*, https://doi.org/10.1016/j.fmre.2025.03.024
51. Li, Y., Lin, T.-y., Luo, Y., Liu, Q., Xiao, W., Guo, W., et al. (2014). A smart and versatile theranostic nanomedicine platform based on nanoporphyrin. *Nature Communications, 5*(1), 4712, https://doi.org/10.1038/ncomms5712.
52. Kemp, J. A., & Kwon, Y. J. (2021). Cancer nanotechnology: current status and perspectives. *Nano Converg, 8*(1), 34, https://doi.org/10.1186/s40580-021-00282-7.

References

53. Wang, C., & Zhang, S. (2023). Advantages of Nanomedicine in Cancer Therapy: A Review. *ACS Applied Nano Materials, 6*(24), 22594–22610, https://doi.org/10.1021/acsanm.3c04487.
54. Hosseini, S. M., Mohammadnejad, J., Salamat, S., Beiram Zadeh, Z., Tanhaei, M., & Ramakrishna, S. (2023). Theranostic polymeric nanoparticles as a new approach in cancer therapy and diagnosis: a review. *Materials Today Chemistry, 29*, 101400, https://doi.org/10.1016/j.mtchem.2023.101400
55. Yenurkar, D., Nayak, M., & Mukherjee, S. (2023). Recent advances of nanocrystals in cancer theranostics. *Nanoscale Adv, 5*(16), 4018-4040, https://doi.org/10.1039/d3na00397c.
56. Joseph, E., & Singhvi, G. (2019). Chapter 4 - Multifunctional nanocrystals for cancer therapy: a potential nanocarrier. In A. M. Grumezescu (Ed.), *Nanomaterials for Drug Delivery and Therapy* (pp. 91–116): William Andrew Publishing.
57. Patel, A., Patel, K., Patel, V., Rajput, M. S., Patel, R., & Rajput, A. (2024). Nanocrystals: an emerging paradigm for cancer therapeutics. *Future Journal of Pharmaceutical Sciences, 10*(1), 4, https://doi.org/10.1186/s43094-024-00579-4.
58. Lhaglham, P., Jiramonai, L., Jia, Y., Huang, B., Huang, Y., Gao, X., et al. (2024). Drug nanocrystals: Surface engineering and its applications in targeted delivery. *iScience, 27*(11), 111185, https://doi.org/10.1016/j.isci.2024.111185.
59. Pardhi, V. P., Verma, T., Flora, S. J. S., Chandasana, H., & Shukla, R. (2018). Nanocrystals: An Overview of Fabrication, Characterization and Therapeutic Applications in Drug Delivery. *Curr Pharm Des, 24*(43), 5129–5146, https://doi.org/10.2174/1381612825666190215121148.
60. Boles, M. A., Ling, D., Hyeon, T., & Talapin, D. V. (2016). The surface science of nanocrystals. *Nature Materials, 15*(2), 141–153, https://doi.org/10.1038/nmat4526.
61. Kang, J., Yang, X., Hu, Q., Cai, Z., Liu, L.-M., & Guo, L. (2023). Recent Progress of Amorphous Nanomaterials. *Chemical Reviews, 123*(13), 8859–8941, https://doi.org/10.1021/acs.chemrev.3c00229.
62. van Blaaderen, A. (2009). Quasicrystals from nanocrystals. *Nature, 461*(7266), 892-893, https://doi.org/10.1038/461892a.
63. Zuo, J. M., & Spence, J. C. H. (2017). Structure of Nanocrystals, Nanoparticles, and Nanotubes. In J. M. Zuo, & J. C. H. Spence (Eds.), *Advanced Transmission Electron Microscopy: Imaging and Diffraction in Nanoscience* (pp. 581–652). New York, NY: Springer New York.
64. Arya, M., Heera, S., Meenu, P., & Deepa, K. G. (2024). Organic-inorganic hybrid materials and architectures in optoelectronic devices: Recent advancements. *ChemPhysMater, 3*(3), 252–272, https://doi.org/10.1016/j.chphma.2024.03.004.
65. Mir, S. H., Nagahara, L. A., Thundat, T., Mokarian-Tabari, P., Furukawa, H., & Khosla, A. (2018). Review—Organic-Inorganic Hybrid Functional Materials: An Integrated Platform for Applied Technologies. *Journal of The Electrochemical Society, 165*(8), B3137, https://doi.org/10.1149/2.0191808jes.
66. Trucillo, P. (2024). Biomaterials for Drug Delivery and Human Applications. *Materials (Basel), 17*(2), https://doi.org/10.3390/ma17020456.
67. Yi, W., Xiao, P., Liu, X., Zhao, Z., Sun, X., Wang, J., et al. (2022). Recent advances in developing active targeting and multi-functional drug delivery systems via bioorthogonal chemistry. *Signal transduction and targeted therapy, 7*(1), 386, https://doi.org/10.1038/s41392-022-01250-1.
68. Manzari, M. T., Shamay, Y., Kiguchi, H., Rosen, N., Scaltriti, M., & Heller, D. A. (2021). Targeted drug delivery strategies for precision medicines. *Nature Reviews Materials, 6*(4), 351–370, https://doi.org/10.1038/s41578-020-00269-6.
69. Jarvis, M., Krishnan, V., & Mitragotri, S. (2019). Nanocrystals: A perspective on translational research and clinical studies. *Bioeng Transl Med, 4*(1), 5–16, https://doi.org/10.1002/btm2.10122.

70. Gressler, S., Hipfinger, C., Part, F., Pavlicek, A., Zafiu, C., & Giese, B. (2025). A systematic review of nanocarriers used in medicine and beyond — definition and categorization framework. *Journal of Nanobiotechnology, 23*(1), 90, https://doi.org/10.1186/s12951-025-03113-7.
71. Shen, S., Wu, Y., Liu, Y., & Wu, D. (2017). High drug-loading nanomedicines: progress, current status, and prospects. *Int J Nanomedicine, 12*, 4085–4109, https://doi.org/10.2147/ijn.S132780.
72. Mali, P., & Sherje, A. P. (2022). Cellulose nanocrystals: Fundamentals and biomedical applications. *Carbohydrate Polymers, 275*, 118668, https://doi.org/10.1016/j.carbpol.2021.118668.
73. Jahangir, M. A., Imam, S. S., Muheem, A., Chettupalli, A., Al-Abbasi, F. A., Nadeem, M. S., et al. (2022). Nanocrystals: Characterization Overview, Applications in Drug Delivery, and Their Toxicity Concerns. *Journal of Pharmaceutical Innovation, 17*(1), 237–248, https://doi.org/10.1007/s12247-020-09499-1.
74. Fan, M., Geng, S., Liu, Y., Wang, J., Wang, Y., Zhong, J., et al. (2018). Nanocrystal Technology as a Strategy to Improve Drug Bioavailability and Antitumor Efficacy for the Cancer Treatment. *Curr Pharm Des, 24*(21), 2416–2424, https://doi.org/10.2174/1381612824666180515154109.
75. Han, X., Xu, K., Taratula, O., & Farsad, K. (2019). Applications of nanoparticles in biomedical imaging. *Nanoscale, 11*(3), 799–819, https://doi.org/10.1039/c8nr07769j.
76. Ho, D., Quake, S. R., McCabe, E. R. B., Chng, W. J., Chow, E. K., Ding, X., et al. (2020). Enabling Technologies for Personalized and Precision Medicine. *Trends Biotechnol, 38*(5), 497–518, https://doi.org/10.1016/j.tibtech.2019.12.021.
77. Rossier, B., Jordan, O., Allémann, E., & Rodríguez-Nogales, C. (2024). Nanocrystals and nanosuspensions: an exploration from classic formulations to advanced drug delivery systems. *Drug Delivery and Translational Research, 14*(12), 3438–3451, https://doi.org/10.1007/s13346-024-01559-0.
78. Romero, G., & Moya, S. E. (2012). Chapter 4 - Synthesis of Organic Nanoparticles. In J. M. de la Fuente, & V. Grazu (Eds.), *Frontiers of Nanoscience* (Vol. 4, pp. 115–141): Elsevier.
79. Yin, R., Tarnsangpradit, J., Gul, A., Jeong, J., Hu, X., Zhao, Y., et al. (2024). Organic nanoparticles with tunable size and rigidity by hyperbranching and cross-linking using microemulsion ATRP. *Proceedings of the National Academy of Sciences, 121*(29), e2406337121, https://doi.org/10.1073/pnas.2406337121.
80. Xiang, H., Xu, S., Li, J., Li, Y., Xue, X., Liu, Y., et al. (2022). Functional drug nanocrystals for cancer-target delivery. *Journal of Drug Delivery Science and Technology, 76*, 103807, https://doi.org/10.1016/j.jddst.2022.103807.
81. Delille, F., Pu, Y., Lequeux, N., & Pons, T. (2022). Designing the Surface Chemistry of Inorganic Nanocrystals for Cancer Imaging and Therapy. *Cancers (Basel), 14*(10), https://doi.org/10.3390/cancers14102456.
82. Sanchis-Gual, R., Coronado-Puchau, M., Mallah, T., & Coronado, E. (2023). Hybrid nanostructures based on gold nanoparticles and functional coordination polymers: Chemistry, physics and applications in biomedicine, catalysis and magnetism. *Coordination Chemistry Reviews, 480*, 215025, https://doi.org/10.1016/j.ccr.2023.215025
83. Ma, D. (2019). Chapter 1 - Hybrid Nanoparticles: An Introduction. In S. Mohapatra, T. A. Nguyen, & P. Nguyen-Tri (Eds.), *Noble Metal-Metal Oxide Hybrid Nanoparticles* (pp. 3–6): Woodhead Publishing.
84. Thorat, N. D., Townley, H. E., Patil, R. M., Tofail, S. A. M., & Bauer, J. (2020). Comprehensive approach of hybrid nanoplatforms in drug delivery and theranostics to combat cancer. *Drug Discovery Today, 25*(7), 1245–1252, https://doi.org/10.1016/j.drudis.2020.04.018

## References

85. Rajora, A. K., Ahire, E. D., Rajora, M., Singh, S., Bhattacharya, J., & Zhang, H. (2024). Emergence and impact of theranostic-nanoformulation of triple therapeutics for combination cancer therapy. *Smart Medicine, 3*(1), e20230035, https://doi.org/10.1002/SMMD.20230035
86. Kowalik, P., Bujak, P., Penkala, M., & Pron, A. (2021). Organic-to-Aqueous Phase Transfer of Alloyed AgInS2-ZnS Nanocrystals Using Simple Hydrophilic Ligands: Comparison of 11-Mercaptoundecanoic Acid, Dihydrolipoic Acid and Cysteine. *Nanomaterials, 11*(4), 843.
87. De Roo, J. (2023). The Surface Chemistry of Colloidal Nanocrystals Capped by Organic Ligands. *Chemistry of Materials, 35*(10), 3781–3792, https://doi.org/10.1021/acs.chemmater.3c00638.
88. Lu, H., Zhang, S., Wang, J., & Chen, Q. (2021). A Review on Polymer and Lipid-Based Nanocarriers and Its Application to Nano-Pharmaceutical and Food-Based Systems. *Front Nutr, 8*, 783831, https://doi.org/10.3389/fnut.2021.783831.
89. Gimeno-Ferrero, R., Valdivia, V., Fernández, I., García-Martín, M. L., & Pernia Leal, M. (2024). Engineering amphiphilic alkenyl lipids for self-assembly in functional hybrid nanostructures. *Scientific Reports, 14*(1), 28887, https://doi.org/10.1038/s41598-024-79917-8.
90. Bajracharya, R., Song, J. G., Patil, B. R., Lee, S. H., Noh, H. M., Kim, D. H., et al. (2022). Functional ligands for improving anticancer drug therapy: current status and applications to drug delivery systems. *Drug Deliv, 29*(1), 1959–1970, https://doi.org/10.1080/10717544.2022.2089296.
91. Ma, Y., Li, Z.-Z., Lin, H., Chen, S., Zhuo, S., & Wang, X.-D. (2022). Advances in organic micro/nanocrystals with tunable physicochemical properties. *Science China Materials, 65*(3), 593–611, https://doi.org/10.1007/s40843-021-1850-1.
92. Alshammari, B. H., Lashin, M. M. A., Mahmood, M. A., Al-Mubaddel, F. S., Ilyas, N., Rahman, N., et al. (2023). Organic and inorganic nanomaterials: fabrication, properties and applications. *RSC Adv, 13*(20), 13735–13785, https://doi.org/10.1039/d3ra01421e.
93. Kambhampati, P. (2021). Nanoparticles, Nanocrystals, and Quantum Dots: What are the Implications of Size in Colloidal Nanoscale Materials? *The Journal of Physical Chemistry Letters, 12*(20), 4769–4779, https://doi.org/10.1021/acs.jpclett.1c00754.
94. Vines, J. B., Yoon, J. H., Ryu, N. E., Lim, D. J., & Park, H. (2019). Gold Nanoparticles for Photothermal Cancer Therapy. *Front Chem, 7*, 167, https://doi.org/10.3389/fchem.2019.00167.
95. Vangijzegem, T., Lecomte, V., Ternad, I., Van Leuven, L., Muller, R. N., Stanicki, D., et al. (2023). Superparamagnetic Iron Oxide Nanoparticles (SPION): From Fundamentals to State-of-the-Art Innovative Applications for Cancer Therapy. *Pharmaceutics, 15*(1), https://doi.org/10.3390/pharmaceutics15010236.
96. Zhao, X., Li, J., Wang, Q., Zhang, Z., Liu, J., Zhang, C., et al. (2023). Recent Progress on High-Z Metal-Based Nanomaterials for Cancer Radiosensitization. *Chinese Journal of Chemistry, 41*(19), 2545–2556, https://doi.org/10.1002/cjoc.202300132
97. Babaye Abdollahi, B., Malekzadeh, R., Pournaghi Azar, F., Salehnia, F., Naseri, A. R., Ghorbani, M., et al. (2021). Main Approaches to Enhance Radiosensitization in Cancer Cells by Nanoparticles: A Systematic Review. *Adv Pharm Bull, 11*(2), 212–223, https://doi.org/10.34172/apb.2021.025.
98. Ren, X., Chen, D., Wang, Y., Li, H., Zhang, Y., Chen, H., et al. (2022). Nanozymes-recent development and biomedical applications. *J Nanobiotechnology, 20*(1), 92, https://doi.org/10.1186/s12951-022-01295-y.
99. Lu, Y., Lv, Y., & Li, T. (2019). Hybrid drug nanocrystals. *Advanced Drug Delivery Reviews, 143*, 115–133, https://doi.org/10.1016/j.addr.2019.06.006.
100. Yaşayan, G., Alarcin, E., Avci-Adali, M., Ipek, T. C., Nejati, O., Özcan-Bülbül, E., et al. (2024). Chapter 27 - Biocompatibility and toxicity challenges of nanomaterials. In H.

Barabadi, E. Mostafavi, & C. Mustansar Hussain (Eds.), *Functionalized Nanomaterials for Cancer Research* (pp. 603–631): Academic Press.
101. Tonelli, F. M. P., Tonelli, F. C. P., Ferreira, D. R. C., Emanuelle da Silva, K., Cordeiro, H. G., Ouchida, A. T., et al. (2020). Chapter 5 - Biocompatibility and Functionalization of Nanomaterials. In N. Ahmad, & P. Gopinath (Eds.), *Intelligent Nanomaterials for Drug Delivery Applications* (pp. 85–103): Elsevier.
102. Kasai, H., Nakanishi, H., Baba, K., & Nishida, K. (2011). Functional Organic Nanocrystals. In Y. Masuda (Ed.), *Nanocrystal*. Rijeka: IntechOpen.
103. Samir, A., Ashour, F. H., Hakim, A. A. A., & Bassyouni, M. (2022). Recent advances in biodegradable polymers for sustainable applications. *npj Materials Degradation, 6*(1), 68, https://doi.org/10.1038/s41529-022-00277-7.
104. Suk, J. S., Xu, Q., Kim, N., Hanes, J., & Ensign, L. M. (2016). PEGylation as a strategy for improving nanoparticle-based drug and gene delivery. *Adv Drug Deliv Rev, 99*(Pt A), 28–51, https://doi.org/10.1016/j.addr.2015.09.012.
105. Barenholz, Y. (2012). Doxil® — The first FDA-approved nano-drug: Lessons learned. *Journal of Controlled Release, 160*(2), 117–134, https://doi.org/10.1016/j.jconrel.2012.03.020.
106. Makadia, H. K., & Siegel, S. J. (2011). Poly Lactic-co-Glycolic Acid (PLGA) as Biodegradable Controlled Drug Delivery Carrier. *Polymers (Basel), 3*(3), 1377–1397, https://doi.org/10.3390/polym3031377.
107. Wang, J., Wang, H., Zou, F., Gu, J., Deng, S., Cao, Y., et al. (2025). The Role of Inorganic Nanomaterials in Overcoming Challenges in Colorectal Cancer Diagnosis and Therapy. *Pharmaceutics, 17*(4), 409.
108. Hu, L., Zhong, H., & He, Z. (2021). Toxicity evaluation of cadmium-containing quantum dots: A review of optimizing physicochemical properties to diminish toxicity. *Colloids and Surfaces B: Biointerfaces, 200*, 111609, https://doi.org/10.1016/j.colsurfb.2021.111609.
109. Le, N., Zhang, M., & Kim, K. (2022). Quantum Dots and Their Interaction with Biological Systems. *Int J Mol Sci, 23*(18), https://doi.org/10.3390/ijms231810763.
110. Medici, S., Peana, M., Pelucelli, A., & Zoroddu, M. A. (2021). An updated overview on metal nanoparticles toxicity. *Seminars in Cancer Biology, 76*, 17–26, https://doi.org/10.1016/j.semcancer.2021.06.020.
111. Raikar, A. S., Priya, S., Bhilegaonkar, S. P., Somnache, S. N., & Kalaskar, D. M. (2023). Surface Engineering of Bioactive Coatings for Improved Stent Hemocompatibility: A Comprehensive Review. *Materials (Basel), 16*(21), https://doi.org/10.3390/ma16216940.
112. Roh, S., Jang, Y., Yoo, J., & Seong, H. (2023). Surface Modification Strategies for Biomedical Applications: Enhancing Cell–Biomaterial Interfaces and Biochip Performances. *BioChip Journal, 17*(2), 174–191, https://doi.org/10.1007/s13206-023-00104-4.
113. Kankala, R. K. (2022). Organic- or Inorganic-based Nanomaterials: Opportunities and Challenges in the Selection for Biomedicines. *Curr Pharm Des, 28*(3), 208–215, https://doi.org/10.2174/1381612827666211007150414.
114. Godja, N. C., & Munteanu, F. D. (2024). Hybrid Nanomaterials: A Brief Overview of Versatile Solutions for Sensor Technology in Healthcare and Environmental Applications. *Biosensors (Basel), 14*(2), https://doi.org/10.3390/bios14020067.
115. Rani, G., & Bala, A. (2022). Chapter 3 - Approaches for synthesis of nanocrystals: an overview. In S. Mallakpour, & C. M. Hussain (Eds.), *Industrial Applications of Nanocrystals* (pp. 43–52): Elsevier.
116. Pelikh, O., Stahr, P.-L., Huang, J., Gerst, M., Scholz, P., Dietrich, H., et al. (2018). Nanocrystals for improved dermal drug delivery. *European Journal of Pharmaceutics and Biopharmaceutics, 128*, 170–178, https://doi.org/10.1016/j.ejpb.2018.04.020.

117. Rashid, A. B., Hoque, M. E., Kabir, N., Rifat, F. F., Ishrak, H., Alqahtani, A., et al. (2023). Synthesis, Properties, Applications, and Future Prospective of Cellulose Nanocrystals. *Polymers (Basel), 15*(20), https://doi.org/10.3390/polym15204070.
118. Tenchov, R., Hughes, K. J., Ganesan, M., Iyer, K. A., Ralhan, K., Lotti Diaz, L. M., et al. (2025). Transforming Medicine: Cutting-Edge Applications of Nanoscale Materials in Drug Delivery. *ACS Nano, 19*(4), 4011–4038, https://doi.org/10.1021/acsnano.4c09566.
119. Wang, W., Zhang, M., Pan, Z., Biesold, G. M., Liang, S., Rao, H., et al. (2022). Colloidal Inorganic Ligand-Capped Nanocrystals: Fundamentals, Status, and Insights into Advanced Functional Nanodevices. *Chemical Reviews, 122*(3), 4091–4162, https://doi.org/10.1021/acs.chemrev.1c00478.
120. Heuer-Jungemann, A., Feliu, N., Bakaimi, I., Hamaly, M., Alkilany, A., Chakraborty, I., et al. (2019). The Role of Ligands in the Chemical Synthesis and Applications of Inorganic Nanoparticles. *Chemical Reviews, 119*(8), 4819–4880, https://doi.org/10.1021/acs.chemrev.8b00733.
121. Namakka, M., Rahman, M. R., Said, K. A. M. B., Abdul Mannan, M., & Patwary, A. M. (2023). A review of nanoparticle synthesis methods, classifications, applications, and characterization. *Environmental Nanotechnology, Monitoring & Management, 20*, 100900, https://doi.org/10.1016/j.enmm.2023.100900.
122. Schauer, D. G., Bredehoeft, J., Yunusa, U., Pattammattel, A., Wörner, H. J., & Sprague-Klein, E. A. (2024). Targeted synthesis of gold nanorods and characterization of their tailored surface properties using optical and X-ray spectroscopy. *Physical Chemistry Chemical Physics, 26*(39), 25581–25589, https://doi.org/10.1039/D4CP01993H.
123. Chen, X., Argandona, S. M., Melle, F., Rampal, N., & Fairen-Jimenez, D. (2024). Advances in surface functionalization of next-generation metal-organic frameworks for biomedical applications: Design, strategies, and prospects. *Chem, 10*(2), 504–543, https://doi.org/10.1016/j.chempr.2023.09.016.
124. Yadav, A., Dogra, P., Sagar, P., Srivastava, M., Srivastava, A., Kumar, R., et al. (2025). A contemporary overview on quantum dots-based fluorescent biosensors: Exploring synthesis techniques, sensing mechanism and applications. *Spectrochimica Acta Part A: Molecular and Biomolecular Spectroscopy, 335*, 126002, https://doi.org/10.1016/j.saa.2025.126002.
125. Jafari, S., Mahyad, B., Hashemzadeh, H., Janfaza, S., Gholikhani, T., & Tayebi, L. (2020). Biomedical Applications of TiO(2) Nanostructures: Recent Advances. *Int J Nanomedicine, 15*, 3447–3470, https://doi.org/10.2147/ijn.S249441.
126. Ghazi, R., Ibrahim, T. K., Nasir, J. A., Gai, S., Ali, G., Boukhris, I., et al. (2025). Iron oxide based magnetic nanoparticles for hyperthermia, MRI and drug delivery applications: a review. *RSC Adv, 15*(15), 11587–11616, https://doi.org/10.1039/d5ra00728c.
127. Wu, J. (2021). The Enhanced Permeability and Retention (EPR) Effect: The Significance of the Concept and Methods to Enhance Its Application. *J Pers Med, 11*(8), https://doi.org/10.3390/jpm11080771.
128. Hussain, Z., Akbari, A. H., Barbuor, S. H., Dawood Alshetiwi, D. S., Ahmed, I. S., & Rawas-Qalaji, M. (2024). Hyaluronic acid based functionalization of nanodelivery systems: A promising strategy for CD44-receptors-mediated targeted therapy of lung cancer. *Journal of Drug Delivery Science and Technology, 101*, 106183, https://doi.org/10.1016/j.jddst.2024.106183.
129. Manzari-Tavakoli, A., Babajani, A., Tavakoli, M. M., Safaeinejad, F., & Jafari, A. (2024). Integrating natural compounds and nanoparticle-based drug delivery systems: A novel strategy for enhanced efficacy and selectivity in cancer therapy. *Cancer Medicine, 13*(5), e7010, https://doi.org/10.1002/cam4.7010.

130. Wang, Z., Deng, X., Ding, J., Zhou, W., Zheng, X., & Tang, G. (2018). Mechanisms of drug release in pH-sensitive micelles for tumour targeted drug delivery system: A review. *International Journal of Pharmaceutics, 535*(1), 253–260, https://doi.org/10.1016/j.ijpharm.2017.11.003.

131. Yi, Z., Yang, X., Liang, Y., & Tong, S. (2024). Iron oxide nanozymes enhanced by ascorbic acid for macrophage-based cancer therapy. *Nanoscale, 16*(30), 14330–14338, https://doi.org/10.1039/D4NR01208A.

132. Feyzizadeh, M., Barfar, A., Nouri, Z., Sarfraz, M., Zakeri-Milani, P., & Valizadeh, H. (2022). Overcoming multidrug resistance through targeting ABC transporters: lessons for drug discovery. *Expert Opin Drug Discov, 17*(9), 1013–1027, https://doi.org/10.1080/17460441.2022.2112666.

133. Gonçalves, A. C., Falcão, A., Alves, G., Lopes, J. A., & Silva, L. R. (2022). Employ of Anthocyanins in Nanocarriers for Nano Delivery: In Vitro and In Vivo Experimental Approaches for Chronic Diseases. *Pharmaceutics, 14*(11), https://doi.org/10.3390/pharmaceutics14112272.

134. Xu, C., Li, S., Chen, J., Wang, H., Li, Z., Deng, Q., et al. (2023). Doxorubicin and erastin co-loaded hydroxyethyl starch-polycaprolactone nanoparticles for synergistic cancer therapy. *Journal of Controlled Release, 356*, 256–271, https://doi.org/10.1016/j.jconrel.2023.03.001.

135. Piccolo, O., Lincoln, J. D., Melong, N., Orr, B. C., Fernandez, N. R., Borsavage, J., et al. (2022). Radiation dose enhancement using gold nanoparticles with a diamond linear accelerator target: a multiple cell type analysis. *Scientific Reports, 12*(1), 1559, https://doi.org/10.1038/s41598-022-05339-z.

136. Inglut, C. T., Sorrin, A. J., Kuruppu, T., Vig, S., Cicalo, J., Ahmad, H., et al. (2020). Immunological and Toxicological Considerations for the Design of Liposomes. *Nanomaterials (Basel), 10*(2), https://doi.org/10.3390/nano10020190.

137. Chen, W., Huang, J., Guo, Y., Wang, X., Lin, Z., Wei, R., et al. (2025). Nanocrystals for Intravenous Drug Delivery: Composition Development, Preparation Methods and Applications in Oncology. *AAPS PharmSciTech, 26*(3), 66, https://doi.org/10.1208/s12249-025-03064-0.

138. Chen, J., & Cong, X. (2023). Surface-engineered nanoparticles in cancer immune response and immunotherapy: Current status and future prospects. *Biomedicine & Pharmacotherapy, 157*, 113998, https://doi.org/10.1016/j.biopha.2022.113998

139. Sun, L., Li, Z., Lan, J., Wu, Y., Zhang, T., & Ding, Y. (2024). Better together: nanoscale co-delivery systems of therapeutic agents for high-performance cancer therapy. *Front Pharmacol, 15*, 1389922, https://doi.org/10.3389/fphar.2024.1389922.

140. Sanchis, T. (2023). Strategies for multidisciplinary research. *Nature Physics, 19*(12), 1736–1737, https://doi.org/10.1038/s41567-023-02277-z.

# Types of Nanocrystals, Synthesis and Properties: Organic Nanocrystals, Inorganic Nanocrystals, Hybrid Nanocrystals

Nanocrystals are solid drug particles that are devoid of carriers and have a size in the nanometer range while maintaining their distinct crystalline structure. They are essential to targeting techniques based on nanotechnology because of their tiny size, which enables both active and passive administration. They additionally provide a high drug content and improved bioavailability for drugs with limited solubility. Organic, inorganic, and hybrid nanocrystals are among the several types that can exist; each has unique characteristics and uses. Usually made from materials like cellulose, organic nanocrystals provide certain synthetic limitations because of their inadequate mechanical and thermal characteristics. Conversely, semiconductors, metals, or magnetic materials can make up inorganic nanocrystals. Compared to organic nanocrystals, they are more hydrophilic, stable, biocompatible, and nontoxic. When various materials with distinct qualities are combined to create a new material with improved or complementary qualities, this is referred to as a hybrid. These elements can be combined to create hybrid nanocrystals. Additionally, compared to other varieties, organic nanocrystals are more often employed and may be used directly for drug administration without the need for other carriers. Furthermore, they provide a particularly intriguing delivery platform because of their very high drug loading (up to almost 100%) and low requirement for organic solvents or solubilizing agents.

## 2.1 Organic Nanocrystals

Highly organized crystalline forms of organic semiconductor materials, organic nanocrystals have special optoelectronic qualities that make them ideal for photocatalytic uses. Their production requires exact control over the morphology, interface structures, and molecular packing; these factors have a direct impact on their charge transfer, light absorption, and catalytic activity [1]. Kasai et al., explained a thorough analysis of the production processes, characteristics, and uses of organic nanocrystals, with a focus on the importance of size control and the strategies employed to attain it. As crystals of organic compounds that are nanometers in size, organic nanocrystals have special optical properties that greatly rely on their size. Particularly when working with heat-sensitive or structurally fragile organic materials, traditional manufacturing procedures like evaporation in inert gas or milling methods have limits and frequently produce crystals that are bigger or less homogeneous in size. The study emphasizes the benefits of the reprecipitation technique, which creates monodispersed nanocrystals with controlled sizes smaller than 50 nm by dissolving organic compounds in a good solvent and then quickly injecting this solution into a poor solvent, such as water. This technique overcomes the limitations of evaporation and works particularly well for organic chemicals that become unstable at high temperatures. Furthermore, sophisticated methods like as supercritical fluid crystallization provide control over size and shape. Crucially, these nanocrystals' optical characteristics, including their absorption and emission spectra, frequently change with size, displaying a phenomenon akin to quantum confinement in which smaller nanocrystals have higher-energy absorption peaks. Opportunities for customized applications in domains including organic photoconductors, pigments, and biological materials are made possible by this size-dependent optical behavior. All things considered, the reprecipitation process is a strong and adaptable method for creating uniformly sized, high-quality organic nanocrystals with adjustable optical characteristics that hold promise for significant industrial uses [2]. The traditional view of carbon nanodots (CNDs) as exclusively carbogenic nanoparticles is being challenged by recent research showing that tiny molecular organic nanocrystals, especially those made from methylenesuccinic acid, display characteristics very similar to CNDs. According to the study, methylenesuccinic acid is created when citric acid is hydrothermally treated. This methylenesuccinic acid then creates hydrogen-bonded nano-assemblies that exhibit properties similar to CND. Fluorescence correlation spectroscopy (FCS) detects the presence of a considerably smaller molecule fluorophore, around 0.9 nm in hydrodynamic diameter, whereas transmission electron microscopy (TEM) frequently displays particles with an average diameter of 3–5 nm. Instead of validating the development of carbogenic CNDs, this contradiction implies that the bigger particles seen by TEM are probably drying-mediated nanocrystals of methylenesuccinic acid. Instead of a carbonized core, these tiny molecular entities and their aggregates, which develop during the drying process, are responsible for the optical characteristics, like excitation-dependent multicolor fluorescence. Based on their optical

## 2.1 Organic Nanocrystals

fingerprints and TEM investigations, many materials that were previously categorized as CNDs may really be molecular fluorophores producing nanocrystalline aggregates.

Thus, a better knowledge of these materials' real structures is essential for the development of CND research, highlighting the necessity of more robust experimental evidence to differentiate genuine carbogenic nanoparticles from organic nanocrystals with comparable optical properties [3]. A type of organic nanocrystals known as Metal–Organic Frameworks (MOFs) is extremely desirable for a variety of applications, including drug administration, catalysis, gas storage, and sensing, due to their exceptional size-dependent functional characteristics. MOF nanocrystals have benefits over their bulk counterparts, including improved guest-sorption kinetics, larger surface-to-volume ratios, and increased bioavailability. However, the consistent production of particles with homogeneous sizes is a major difficulty in this sector. The majority of MOF materials have not been effectively synthesized as nanocrystals, but several have, and the common nano-MOF sizes are typically in the range of 100–20 nm. For MOF nanocrystals to be tailored to particular applications, exact control over their size is essential. Understanding the kinetic rivalry between metal–ligand reactivity and acid–base reactivity during nanocrystal development allows for this control. The nature and amount of modulators, the linker or modulator equivalents, and the metal–ligand bond strengths are important factors that affect nano-MOF sizes. When ligands outcompete metal-ion transport, resulting in kinetically confined particle sizes, the formation of these nanocrystals stops. A suggested 'seesaw' connection provides a roadmap for exact synthetic control by illustrating the link between nanocrystal sizes and acidic surface-capping ligand concentrations. Depleting local concentrations of reactant metal ions is ultimately necessary to achieve tiny MOF nanocrystal sizes, which enables linkers and monotopic modulators to trap the particles [4]. Over the past three decades, metal–organic frameworks (MOFs), a noteworthy family of porous crystalline materials, have attracted a lot of interest in the adsorption sector (Fig. 2.1). A metal cluster (also known as a secondary building unit, or SBU) and organic linkers, that join the metal clusters to create 1D, 2D, or 3D periodic network designs, are the two main building pieces that make up these materials. MOFs have a number of qualities, including as high, permanent porosities and very wide surface areas, which make them great options for adsorption applications. These characteristics are essential for pollutants to effectively diffuse into the porous network and reach the adsorption sites. Furthermore, by carefully choosing metal clusters and organic linkers, MOFs may be dynamically built to adjust their surface area, pore size and shape, and the kind and concentration of their adsorption sites. The strength and kind of relationships among the MOF structure and the pollutants are determined by this control at the adsorption sites, which is crucial since it affects the adsorption's selectivity and capacity [5]. With their distinct optical and electrical characteristics, organic nanocrystals, nanoscale crystalline formations made of organic molecules, are extremely advantageous for a variety of applications, especially in the domains of photonics and optoelectronics. Since triplet–triplet energy transfer is essential for efficient energy storage and delivery in organic photoelectric materials, these nanocrystals can be designed to improve light-harvesting efficiency. Novel methods in solar energy conversion, lighting, and display systems have been made possible by recent developments in the manufacturing and analysis of organic nanocrystals, which have produced bright organic nanocrystals for applications in biology and light-harvesting systems that imitate natural processes [6]. Because of their distinct and well-organized molecular configurations, organic nanocrystals are nanoscale crystalline solids made solely of organic molecules. These nanocrystals' high surface-to-volume ratios and quantum confinement effects result in distinctive optical, electrical, and mechanical characteristics that set them apart from their bulk counterparts. They are very appealing for use in optoelectronic devices such light-emitting diodes, lasers, sensors, and bio-imaging because of their tiny size and crystallinity, which allow for improved light absorption, emission, and charge transfer. Their optical characteristics, including as stability, quantum yield, and emission wavelength, may be tuned thanks to the exact control over size and shape during synthesis. Additionally, organic nanocrystals frequently exhibit enhanced ability to process and suitability with flexible substrates, which makes it easier to incorporate them into the adaptive and lightweight electronic gadgets of the future. As shown in the study under discussion, pressure-induced structural changes greatly increased the white-light emission of MOF nanocrystals. Recent developments have concentrated on enhancing their stability and luminescent efficiency through surface passivation, pressure treatments, and structural modifications.

Organic nanocrystals are a viable foundation for creating cutting-edge functional materials for biomedical technology, sustainable lighting, and displays because of their

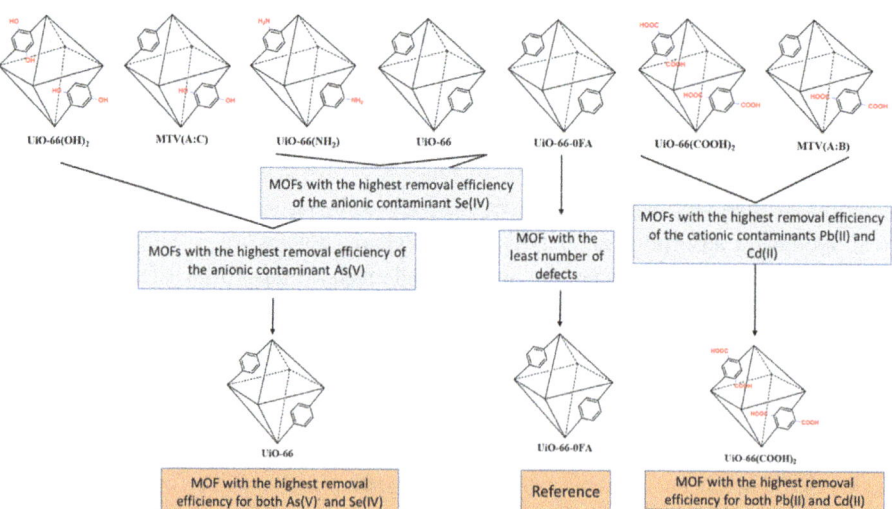

**Fig. 2.1** Pb(II), Cd(II), As(V), and Se(IV) adsorption flow chart showing the Screening of the Various UiO-66-Based Structures

adaptability and adjustable qualities [7]. Known for their remarkable chiroptical qualities, biocompatibility, sustainability, and ease of processing, organic nanocrystals in particular, cellulose nanocrystals, or CNCs are adaptable nanoscale building blocks (Fig. 2.2). These nanocrystals can self-assemble forming left-handed chiral photonic frameworks with a one-dimensional photonic bandgap and have a twisted morphology that comes from individual molecules. They are able to convert spontaneous luminescence into circularly polarized luminescence and split incident light onto circularly polarized reflected and transmitted light thanks to their special self-assembly. Techniques like ultrasonication, which disassembles aggregates and alters particle shape, can have an impact on the creation of these structures and alter the film reflection band. The production of near-infrared circularly polarized light for cancer diagnosis, bioimaging, biotherapy, and quantum communication methods are just a few of the cutting-edge uses for organic nanocrystals, particularly CNC films. High luminescence dissymmetry factors and resolving problems like structural flaws and luminescence intensity heterogeneity, that might impair their performance, are still difficult to achieve [8].

## 2.2 Inorganic Nanocrystals

The adjustable optical characteristics, exceptional photothermal and photodynamic transition efficiencies, and good biocompatibility of inorganic nanocrystals, especially light-responsive ones, make them a revolutionary frontier in biomedical engineering [9, 10]. These substances, which include gold-based nanostructures, graphite carbon nitride, transitional metal oxides, up conversion nanoparticles, and carbon-based nanomaterials (such as graphene and carbon nanotubes), are designed to react to particular light wavelengths, particularly in the near-infrared spectrum, to initiate therapeutic or diagnostic processes like specific drug delivery, cancer cell ablation, and regenerative stimulation [11]. Applications like photodynamic therapy (PDT), photothermal therapy (PTT), non-genetic optical modulation of cells, and the development of remote-controlled drug delivery systems and actuators are made possible by their special capacity to transform light into heat, chemical energy, or electrical signals. For instance, specific surface plasmon resonance in gold nanorods results in good photothermal effects, while hydrogels based on graphene oxide may dynamically modify stiffness to affect cellular activity and encourage wound healing [12, 13]. The higher photostability, more deep tissue penetration, and multifunctionalization capabilities of inorganic nanocrystals over organic photosensitizers make them essential to next-generation medical technologies targeted at personalized medicine and less invasive therapies [14]. The nonlinear optical characteristics of inorganic nanocrystals, notably all-inorganic perovskite nanocrystals like $CsPbBr_3$, and their promise for enhanced biomedical imaging, particularly multiphoton bioimaging, have attracted a lot of attention. These nanocrystals are ideal for deep-tissue imaging with little photodamage because of their remarkable multiphoton absorption cross-sections,

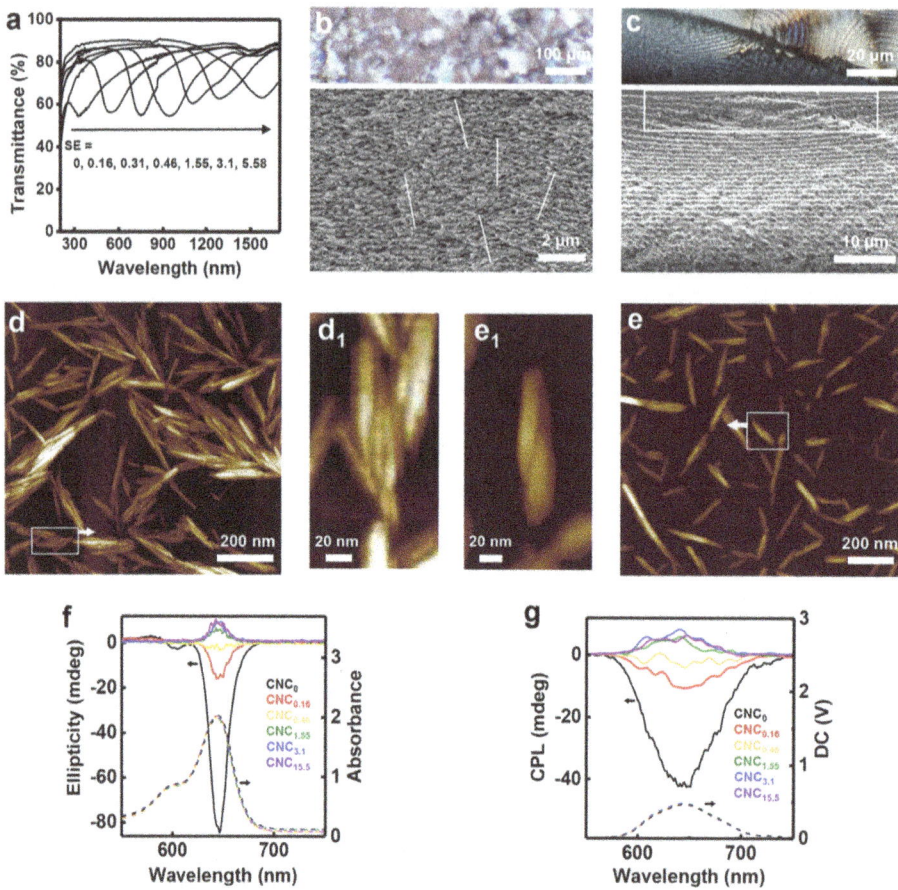

**Fig. 2.2** Chirality of CNCSE and characterization of CNCSE-λ films. **a** As sonication energy increases, red-shifted reflection bands are seen in the transmission spectra of CNCSE-λ. **b** and **c** SEM (bottom) and POM (top) pictures demonstrate the development of chiral photonics polydomains (white lines) in CNC0.38–780 and a bilayer film with a bottom layer of planar anchored chiral photonics and a top layer of focal conics (white rectangle) in CNC10-2100. **d, e** There are more bound bundles in CNC0 as well as additional nanorod bundles in CNC15.5 (e, e1), according to AFM pictures. **f** The CNCSE/Cy5-NHS solutions' sonication-energy-dependent circular dichroism patterns are seen in the circular dichroism spectra (aq.). **g** The CP luminescence spectra of the CNCSE/CdSe-ZnS solutions (aq.) display sonication-energy-dependent CP luminescence signals

adjustable emission spectra, and robust photoluminescence. However, their biological uses have been limited due to their intrinsic fragility in aquatic settings. By encasing $CsPbBr_3$ nanocrystals in a silica ($SiO_2$) shell and then incorporating them in PEGylated phospholipid micelles (mPEG-DSPE), this team overcame that difficulty and produced

## 2.2 Inorganic Nanocrystals

water-dispersible, photostable, and biocompatible nanocrystals. These hybrid nanostructures exhibited minimal cytotoxicity across a variety of cell lines, maintained stability under extreme circumstances including UV exposure and ultrasonication, and displayed strong photoluminescence with 1,2,3-photon excitation. Furthermore, folic acid (FA) functionalization improved targeted uptake in cancer cells that expressed the folate receptor, hence facilitating their application in accurate cellular imaging. The construction of stable, nontoxic inorganic nanocrystal platforms for deep-tissue, high-resolution, targeted image analysis in biomedical research and diagnostics is generally advanced by our discoveries [15]. The unique photoluminescent features and biocompatibility of inorganic nanocrystals, especially those created by surface-functionalized combination systems like europium(III) complex-based hydroxyapatite (EHA), provide increased possibilities for quick and precise cancer cell imaging. Using amplification of folate receptors, EHA nanocrystals were created in this work by combining the Eu(III) complex with hydroxyapatite and then modifying it with folic acid (FA) derivatives to target HeLa cancer cells specifically. Low occupancy (~3–5%) exhibits the maximum quantum efficiency and red luminescence because of the effective charge-transfer interactions between FA-NHS and EuTH. The molecular population of FA-NHS on the nanocrystal surface was adjusted to maximize luminescence efficiency and targeting ability.

These nanohybrids maintained good cell viability at different doses by exhibiting minimal cytotoxicity, great dispersibility under physiological settings, and outstanding photostability. Furthermore, they are perfect candidates for quick, non-invasive imaging due to their quick entry into cells and high fluorescence when excited optically. With intriguing potential for real-time cancer diagnostics and photonic biomedical applications, this is a major advance in the creation of multifunctional inorganic nanocrystals that combine selective cellular uptake, biosafety, and efficient luminous output [16]. The outstanding photoluminescence, quantum yield, and nonlinear optical features of inorganic nanocrystals, especially cesium lead halide perovskites ($CsPbBr_3$), have shown great promise as next-generation bioimaging probes. By merely altering the water volume, a unique water-triggered synthesis technique was created to transform non-emissive 0D $CsPbBr_6$ into very stable and biocompatible 1D nanowires, 2D nanoplatelets, and 3D nanocubes of $CsPbBr_3$. These nanocrystals demonstrated exceptional photostability, retaining over 85% of their luminescence after 35 days in water and 99% after extended UV exposure (Fig. 2.3). They were encapsulated with polyethylene glycol (PEG) for improved water dispersibility and biocompatibility. Their remarkable two-photon absorption (2PA) cross-sections were orders of magnitude greater than those of traditional organic fluorophores, allowing for high-resolution, deep-tissue imaging. HER-2 positive and triple-negative breast cancer (TNBC) cells may be selectively labeled and imaged simultaneously using two-photon technology thanks to antibody conjugation of 1D and 2D nanocrystals. The stability, brightness, and specificity of shape-engineered, PEG-coated $CsPbBr_3$ nanocrystals are much better than those of conventional fluorescent dyes, making them excellent multiphoton imaging agents for biomedical diagnostics

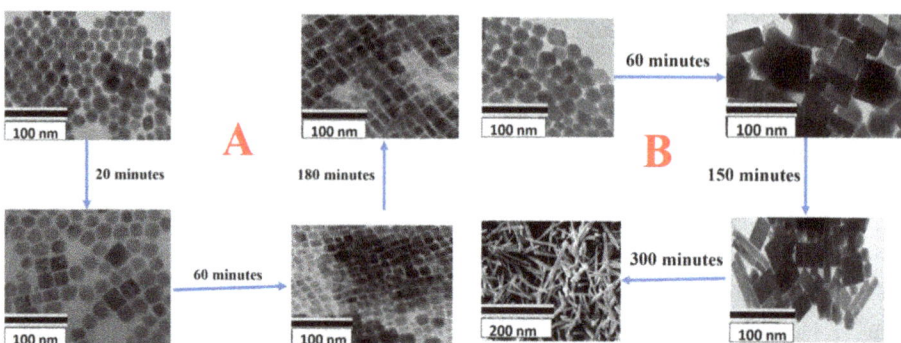

**Fig. 2.3 a** The transformation of Cs4PbBr$_6$ NCs to 2D CsPbBr$_3$ nanoplatelets by self-organization during water-triggered synthesis is demonstrated by time-dependent TEM image data. **b** The transformation of Cs4PbBr$_6$ NCs to 1D CsPbBr$_3$ nanowires via self-organization during water-triggered synthesis is demonstrated by time-dependent TEM image data

[17]. For near-infrared (NIR) photodynamic treatment (PDT), inorganic nanocrystals are becoming powerful photosensitizers, especially in the understudied NIR-III window (1350–1870 nm).

This work shows that under 1567 nm laser irradiation, acid-etching CoMo-LDH and NiMo-LDH nanosheets creates oxygen vacancies and changes their electronic band structures, significantly increasing their capacity to produce reactive oxygen species (ROS), including singlet oxygen ($^1O_2$). These defect-rich LDHs (DR-CoMo-LDH, for example) efficiently promote tumor ablation and cancer cell death both in vitro and in vivo, and they produce ROS at a rate that is about 97 times greater than that of their pristine counterparts. Polyethylene glycol (PEG) surface modification guarantees superior stability, tumor-targeting ability, and biocompatibility. Furthermore, by breaking down $H_2O_2$ in the tumor microenvironment, these nanocrystals can stimulate the synthesis of oxygen, overcoming hypoxia, a significant obstacle in PDT. Notably, DR-CoMo-LDH nanosheets have low toxicity and deep tissue penetration, opening the door for low-invasive, highly effective cancer treatment platforms that use inorganic nanocrystals in the NIR-III range [18]. With regulated degradability to reduce nanotoxicity, inorganic nanocrystals in particular, manganese oxide nanoparticles, or MNPs have been developed for multipurpose cancer theranostics, providing both therapeutic and diagnostic properties (Fig. 2.4). MONPs were surface-modified in this work using EDTA and bovine serum albumin (BSA) to improve their safety, water dispersibility, and biocompatibility. They also functioned as dual-mode MRI contrast agents and efficient PTT agents. Importantly, ascorbic acid may be used to intentionally induce their breakdown, giving precision control over their breakdown into excretable, non-toxic metabolites like $Mn^{2+}$ ions, which are then further trapped by BSA and EDTA to avoid systemic toxicity. In comparison to gold nanorods, these nanocrystals exhibit higher performance, high photothermal conversion rate (34.7%), and robust near-infrared (NIR) absorption. Tests conducted in vivo verified the following: low cytotoxicity, even after destruction, limited accumulation in organs, quick clearance, efficient tumor ablation, and tumor targeting. Furthermore, under regulated settings, MONPs may effectively load and release therapeutic medicines, which makes them attractive options for imaging-guided cancer treatment platforms and tailored drug delivery with lower long-term hazards [19].

## 2.3 Hybrid Nanocrystals

Hybrid nanocrystals, often referred to as multifunctional nanocrystals, are a cutting-edge type of nanomedicines intended to carry out both therapeutic and diagnostic tasks concurrently, a process known as "theranostics" in the treatment of cancer. Pure drug nanocrystals, which provide about 100% drug loading, are usually coupled with functional elements like imaging agents, magnetic particles, or targeting ligands to create these structures. While surface modifications such as PEGylation or antibody conjugation allow active targeting to certain tumor cell receptors, their nanoscale size allows passive tumor targeting through the increased permeability and retention (EPR) effect. Hybrid nanocrystals, as opposed to conventional nanoparticle formulations, contain fewer excipients, which lowers toxicity concerns and streamlines regulatory approval. Their crystalline structure, which is physically stable, increases the bioavailability of poorly soluble chemotherapeutics like doxorubicin and paclitaxel, prolongs systemic circulation, and prevents protein binding.

Furthermore, for real-time imaging and tracking of tumor growth or treatment response, hybrid systems can integrate MRI contrast agents or fluorescent dyes. Dual-mode imaging, pH-responsive drug release, and tumor-specific hyperthermia are further made possible by innovations like ceria-based systems or dumbbell-shaped $FeO_4/MnO$ crystals. Despite their potential, problems with controlled release, large-scale production, dosage optimization, and clinical safety still exist. However, hybrid nanocrystals, which provide a single platform for targeted administration, imaging, and treatment, represent the future of personalized oncology [20]. Hybrid nanocrystals are a cutting-edge class of multipurpose nanomaterials that combine the advantages of inorganic and organic components to solve important drug delivery issues (Fig. 2.5). By encasing bupivacaine nanocrystals in thermoresponsive nanogels made of oligo(ethylene glycol) methyl ether methacrylate (OEGMA)-based polymers and then embellishing them with copper sulfide (CuS) nanoparticles that absorb near-infrared (NIR) light, Alejo et al. created a novel hybrid system. A highly effective and externally controlled drug delivery platform is made possible by this hybrid design. In comparison to conventional nanoparticle formulations, the nanocrystals guarantee a high drug loading (up to 65.5 wt%) while preserving the

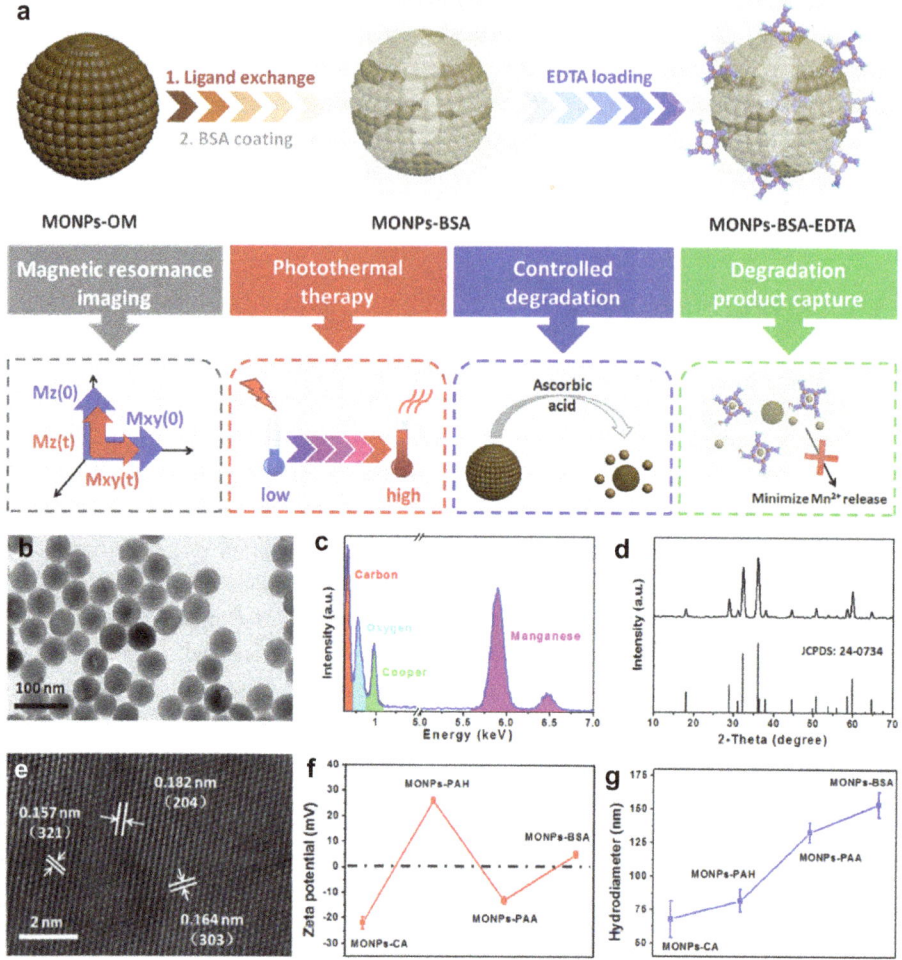

**Fig. 2.4** The basis and description of MONPs-BSA-EDTA. **a** A diagram showing the creation, use, regulated breakdown, and product harvest of multifunctional MONPs-BSA-EDTA. TEM picture (**b**), MONPs-BSA-EDTA's EDXA spectrum (**c**), XRD pattern (**d**), and HR-TEM image (**e**). The hydrodiameter (**g**) and zeta potential (**f**) of MONPs in DI water following each surface coating stage. The relative deviations of the zeta potential and particle size measurements were both less than 0.05

drug in a stable crystalline state for extended release. The CuS nanoparticles' absorption of NIR light causes localized heating in the thermoresponsive polymer matrix, which enables precise, on-demand drug release in both space and time. The collapse of the nanogel caused by this photothermal activation effectively pushes out the medication when needed, which is especially useful for applications like long-term pain treatment where varied dosage is favorable. Crucially, across a variety of cell lines, the hybrid nanocrystals showed outstanding cytocompatibility, indicating their potential for therapeutic application. Overall, the combination of photothermal agents, stimuli-responsive polymers, and nanocrystals in a single nanosystem shows how hybrid nanocrystals can overcome the drawbacks of traditional delivery methods by providing external control over drug administration, sustained release, and high loading efficiency [21]. A potential family of multifunctional materials, hybrid nanocrystals combine the special qualities of several inorganic components in a synergistic way to improve performance in biological applications, especially cancer theranostics. One notable example is the Prussian Blue/Manganese Dioxide (PBMn) hybrid nanocrystal created by Hao et al., which is intended for tumor oxygen management, photothermal treatment (PTT), and trimodal imaging (photoacoustic, T1- and T2-weighted MRI). The one-pot method used to create these nanocrystals involves generating $MnO_2$ in situ from $KMnO_4$ and incorporating it into the Prussian Blue (PB) framework. This results in uniform, monodisperse nanoparticles that are smaller than 50 nm, which is a size that is advantageous for passive tumor targeting through the enhanced permeability and retention (EPR) effect. In addition to regulating the particle size and MRI magnetic characteristics, $MnO_2$ also improves catalytic efficiency in the breakdown of hydrogen peroxide to oxygen, which alleviates tumor hypoxia. Simultaneously, the PB component provides substantial near-infrared (NIR) absorption for effective PTT and functions as a photoacoustic imaging contrast agent. Because of their versatility, PBMn nanocrystals can serve as a "one-for-all" theranostic platform, providing targeted thermal ablation of tumors, active tumor oxygenation to improve MRI contrast and treatment results, and deep-tissue imaging guiding. The possibilities for clinical translation as intelligent nanotheranostic agents is highlighted by their biodegradability, stability under physiological settings, and shown tumor suppression activity in vivo [22]. A new family of multifunctional materials called hybrid nanocrystals combines inorganic and organic components to provide specialized biological and physicochemical properties for cutting-edge biomedical applications. By integrating the luminescent tris(2,2,6,6-tetramethyl-3,5-heptanedionato) europium (III) (EuTH) complex within the HA matrix and altering the surface with folic acid $N$-hydroxysuccinimidyl ester (FA-NHS), a ligand that targets cancer, Kataoka et al. were able to create hybrid nanostructures (EHA) from europium(III) complex-based hydroxyapatite (HA) nanocrystals. The synergistic improvements in photophysical and biological performance were made possible by this special inorganic–organic mix. The FA-NHS provided preferential affinity for HeLa cancer cells through folate receptor-mediated endocytosis, whereas the EuTH provided intense red luminescence with abrupt f–f transitions typical of europium ions. In order to optimize the charge-transfer interactions at the nanohybrid interface and achieve the greatest luminescence quantum efficiency at a $\sim$3% FA-NHS surface occupancy, the FA-NHS density was regulated via surface engineering using silane linkers. With real-time imaging under fluorescent microscopy, the resultant EHA nanohybrids showed outstanding dispersibility in phosphate-buffered saline, non-cytotoxicity, and quick absorption by cancer cells. High signal intensity and specificity for cancer cell imaging are made possible by this design, which also serves as an example of how meticulous control of interfacial molecular interactions in hybrid nanocrystals may result in photofunctional bioimaging agents with adjustable and improved performance [16].

Advanced multifunctional platforms known as hybrid nanocrystals have shown considerable potential in cancer theranostics by combining therapeutic and diagnostic functions into a single nanosystem. Shen et al.'s work presents luminescent/magnetic PLGA-based hybrid nanocomposites designed to deliver vascular endothelial growth factor (VEGF) shRNA and the chemotherapeutic medication doxorubicin (DOX) simultaneously for a synergistic anticancer impact. Within a biodegradable PLGA matrix, these nanocrystals incorporate DOX for chemotherapy, superparamagnetic $FeO_4$ nanoparticles for magnetic resonance imaging (MR), and CdSe/ZnS quantum dots for fluorescence imaging. Polyethyleneimine–polyethylene glycol–folic acid (PEI-PEG-FA) surface engineering improves tumor targeting via both magnetic and folate receptor-mediated mechanisms. To combat tumor angiogenesis, VEGF shRNA is also electrostatically adsorbed onto the surface to silence genes. The hybrid nanocrystals exhibit strong cytotoxicity against cancer cells, high drug-loading efficiency, pH-sensitive release behavior, and superior biocompatibility (Fig. 2.6). With high $T_2$-weighted MR and fluorescence signals both in vitro and in vivo, they demonstrate dual-modality imaging capabilities and effectively suppress tumor development with no systemic damage. These findings highlight the promise of these hybrid nanocrystals as intelligent, multipurpose delivery systems for accurate, image-guided, and focused cancer treatment [23]. The interplay between their organic and inorganic components intimately governs the structural and optoelectronic characteristics of hybrid nanocrystals, especially organic–inorganic halide perovskite nanocrystals (PNCs). The work by Debnath et al. investigates the effects of halide substitution on vibrational coherence and lattice anharmonicity using formamidinium lead halide nanocrystals ($FAPbX_3$, where X = Br or I). Upon ultrafast photoexcitation, these hybrid nanocrystals display significant coherent phonon oscillations, exposing unique vibrational wave packets that are strongly influenced by the halide composition. Modulating the phonon dynamics is largely dependent on the interaction between the inorganic $PbX_6^{4-}$ octahedral cage and the core formamidinium (FA) cation. Specifically, compared to bromide-based nanocrystals ($FAPbBr_3$), iodide-based ones ($FAPbI_3$) exhibit more anharmonic vibrational behavior and greater harmonic production, suggesting weaker $FA-PbI_6$ contacts and a more flexible inorganic lattice. They results are confirmed by theoretical calculations, which show that the FA moiety in iodide lattices has lower rotational energy barriers and that they are associated with higher anharmonic coupling. This lattice anharmonicity affects charge-carrier dynamics and stability by facilitating energy transfer into overtone and combination vibrational bands. Understanding hybrid nanocrystals' halide- and cation-dependent vibrational activity is essential for maximizing their photophysical characteristics and preparing them for use in light-emitting devices, photovoltaics, and other optoelectronic technologies

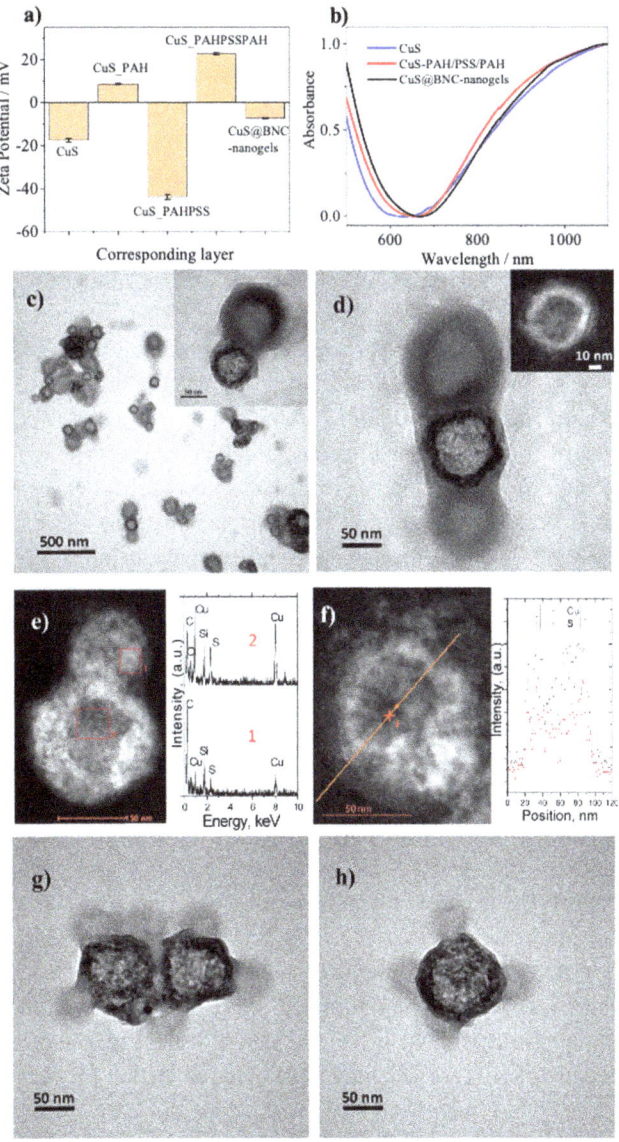

**Fig. 2.5** a Zeta potential by alternating polyelectrolyte adsorption and coupling to BNC-nanogels during CuS NPs LbL coating. b CuS, CuS-PAH/PSS/PAH, and CuS@BNC-nanogels' UV–Vis spectra. CuS@BNC-nanogels in a representative TEM picture (c, d). A detailed HAADF-STEM picture of a CuS nanoparticle is shown in the inset in. CuS nanoparticles' EDS spectra and HAADF-STEM image (e); a typical CuS nanoparticle's Cu/S EDS profiles and HAADF-STEM picture (f). The spatial localization of the EDS profile is shown by the red line in the picture. TEM pictures of empty CuS@nanogels (g, h)

[24]. Because of their exceptional optoelectronic qualities, biocompatibility, and adaptability in biological applications, hybrid nanocrystals especially those made of inorganic/ organic materials are transforming photoelectrochemical (PEC) biosensing. Using L-cysteine-modified Ag–ZnIn$_2$S$_4$ quantum dots (L-Cys AZIS QDs) hybridized with iron phthalocyanine (FePc) to create a Z-scheme photoactive system, Wang et al. created a new PEC cytosensor. By efficiently segregating photogenerated charge carriers, this hybrid arrangement increases photo-to-electric conversion efficiency and greatly improves light absorption in the near-infrared (NIR) spectrum. In addition to increasing solubility and decreasing toxicity, the L-Cys AZIS QDs act as anchors for biological recognition components such hyaluronic acid (HA), which binds the CD44 receptor that is expressed on the membranes of cancer cells. This hybrid nanocrystal system exhibits robust PEC responses under NIR light irradiation, which are significantly diminished following target cell attachment, allowing for label-free, ultrasensitive cancer cell detection. With a wide dynamic range and a low detection limit of 15 cells/mL, the PEC cytosensor has outstanding analytical performance and can effectively distinguish between different cancer cell lines' levels of CD44 expression. This work demonstrates the enormous potential of hybrid nanocrystals in biomedical diagnostics, namely in creating extremely sensitive, non-invasive systems for real-time cancer biomarker monitoring [25]. Researchers can develop multifunctional platforms with improved surface area, conductivity, and biocompatibility by combining materials like reduced graphene oxide (rGO), metal-protein nanostructures like Ag@bovine serum albumin (Ag@BSA), carboxylated carbon nanotubes (CNTs-COOH), and conductive polymers like PEDOT. Protein-templated metal nanostructures provide biocompatibility and catalytic activity, while carbon nanomaterials enable high electron mobility and functional surface chemistry. These composites take use of the special synergy between their organic and inorganic constituents. PEDOT significantly improves the system's electrical characteristics and environmental stability. As evidenced by the accurate identification of carcinoembryonic antigen (CEA), a crucial cancer biomarker, the resultant nanohybrid structures not only facilitate strong antibody immobilization but also improve signal sensitivity and lower detection limits. These nanohybrids frequently perform on par with or better than traditional tests like ELISA, achieving exceptional selectivity, stability, and repeatability in actual blood samples. Hybrid nanocrystals are therefore a possible foundation for next-generation diagnostic tools that may find use in clinical diagnostics and early illness detection [26]. By combining the therapeutic benefits of both organic and inorganic components into a single nanosystem, hybrid nanocrystals like those created by functionalizing paclitaxel (PTX) nanocrystals with silver nanoparticles (AgNPs) and tumor-targeting peptides offer a very promising approach to cancer therapy (Fig. 2.7). In this study, PTX nanocrystals were first made and then coated with polydopamine (PDA), a versatile biopolymer that serves as a stabilizer, reducing agent, and platform for additional modifications. AgNPs were in situ deposited onto the PDA layer, offering additional anti-cancer activity and the ability to tackle drug resistance, while the tumor-targeting NR1 peptide (containing

## 2.3 Hybrid Nanocrystals

the RGD motif) was transferred to enhance specific cellular uptake via αvβ3 integrin interaction. Because of the combined activities of PTX and AgNPs, these multifunctional nanocrystals show synergistic cytotoxicity, pH-responsive drug release, and considerably increased internalization of cancer cells. Additionally, despite retaining superior selectivity and biocompatibility in healthy cells, they exhibit potent pro-apoptotic activity through mitochondrial malfunction, ROS production, and DNA damage.

When taken as a whole, these hybrid nanocrystals offer a unique, carrier-free, tumor-targeted platform that addresses major drawbacks of conventional chemotherapy by optimizing drug delivery effectiveness, therapeutic efficacy, and biosafety [27]. Similarly, AgNP-adorned camptothecin (CPT) nanocrystals provide a potent and complementary method of combating multidrug resistance in cancer treatment. CPT nanocrystals function as a strong chemotherapeutic agent in this formulation, while AgNPs increase cytotoxicity by blocking drug resistance mechanisms such as P-glycoprotein (Pgp) production and activity. When compared to free CPT or naked nanocrystals, the CPT/Ag hybrid nanocrystals show better stability, dispersion, and cellular uptake. Because of their pH-responsive release, CPT and AgNPs are released quickly and precisely into the acidic

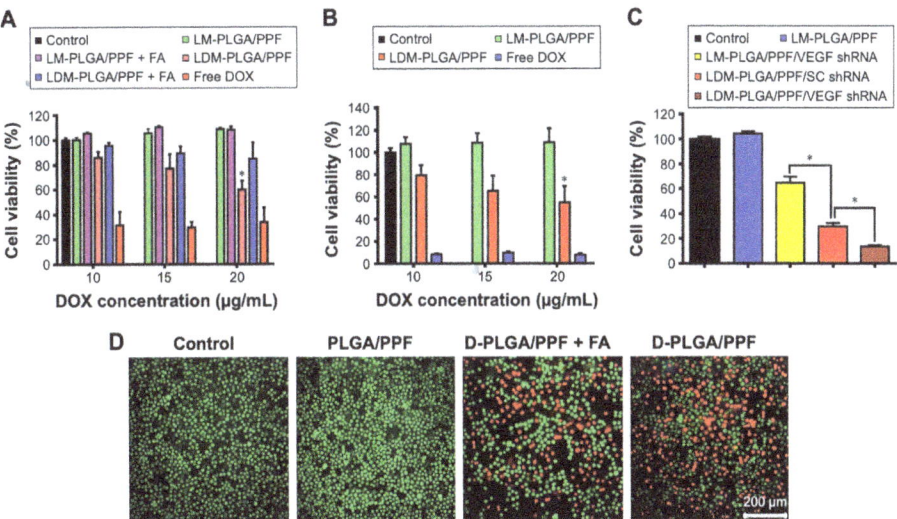

**Fig. 2.6** HeLa (**a**) and EMT-6 (**b**) cells treated with free DOX, LDM Plga/PPF, and LM-Plga/PPF at varying DOX concentrations for 48 h, either with or without a preincubation with free folic acid (1.25 mM), were tested for in vitro cell viability. **c** LDM-PLGA/PPF/VEGF shRNA nanocomposites' synergistic therapeutic effectiveness against EMT-6 cells at a dose of 25 µg/mL of DOX for 72 h. **d** Fluorescence microscopy pictures of HeLa cells stained with calcein-AM and propidium iodide following different treatments at a DOX dosage of 20 µg/mL. Red and green stand for dead and living cells, respectively. *P, 0.05. PPF stands for PEI-PEG-FA; PEI-PEG-FA stands for polyethyleneimine premodified with polyethylene glycol-folic acid; VegF stands for vascular endothelial growth factor; DOX stands for doxorubicin; and Plga for poly(d,l-lactic-co-glycolic acid)

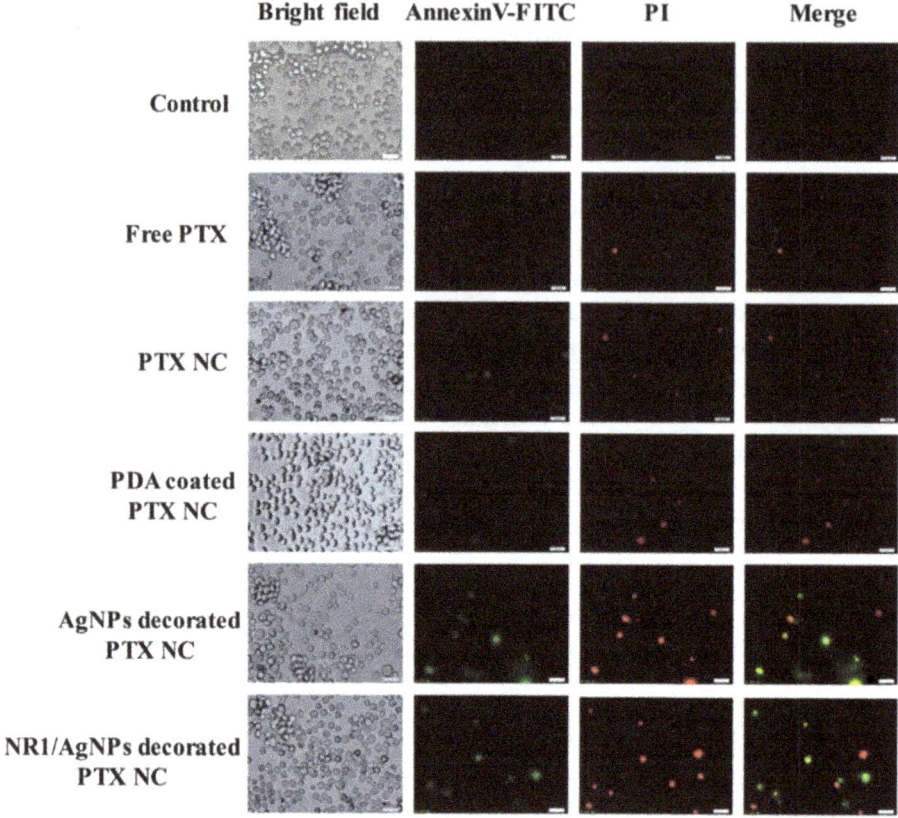

**Fig. 2.7** Fluorescent pictures demonstrating how various PTX formulations affect MDA-MB-231 cells labeled with Annexin V-FITC/PI in terms of cell apoptosis and necrosis. 20 μm is the scale bar

tumor microenvironment. Bypassing efflux pumps and administering high intracellular drug concentrations, this "escape and attack" process causes DNA damage and apoptosis, which are then brought on by successively released CPT and AgNPs. Crucially, these nanocrystals exhibit substantial cytotoxicity against a range of drug-sensitive and drug-resistant tumor cell lines while having no impact on healthy cells, underscoring their potential and therapeutic selectivity. High repeatability and adaptability for additional hydrophobic medicines are guaranteed by the simple and environmentally friendly synthesis using polydopamine-mediated AgNP deposition. All things considered, these hybrid nanocrystals offer a cutting-edge multipurpose platform for effective and focused cancer treatment [28]. Platelet membrane-cloaked paclitaxel nanocrystals (PPNCs), in particular, are a novel drug delivery method that combines the biomimetic targeting ability of platelet membranes with the high drug-loading capacity of nanocrystals to improve postoperative chemotherapy. PEG-PTX intermediate layer enhances hydrophilicity and

## 2.3 Hybrid Nanocrystals

compatibility, a solid paclitaxel nanocrystal (PNC) core delivers high drug doses, and an outer shell made from platelet membranes mimics natural biological interactions to allow for accurate delivery to surgical coagulation locations or tumor-induced bleeding areas. In comparison to uncoated nanocrystals, the PPNCs exhibited improved cellular uptake and cytotoxicity against 4T1 breast cancer cells in addition to outstanding in vitro stability, prolonged drug release, and retention of important membrane proteins. When combined with vascular disrupting drugs such as DMXAA to produce specific coagulation cues, PPNCs effectively accumulated at malignancies or resection sites in vivo, improving treatment effectiveness and extending longevity in mouse breast cancer models. Crucially, PPNCs avoided platelet activation or aggregation, eliminated off-target effects, and decreased systemic toxicity, highlighting their therapeutic promise and biosafety. Thus, this hybrid nanocrystal platform offers a viable and efficient method for administering high-dose, site-specific chemotherapy, particularly in cases of bleeding tumors or postoperative conditions [29]. Similarly, aggregation-induced emission (AIE) fluorophores such as tetraphenylethene (TPE) combined with paclitaxel (PTX) nanocrystals provide a sophisticated method for monitoring intracellular drug breakdown and improving cancer treatment at the same time. Real-time monitoring of the destiny of nanocrystals inside cells is made possible by the physical doping of these hybrid systems with AIE molecules, which glow only when they are confined in motion within the crystalline structure and lose their fluorescence upon disintegration. According to the study, cancer cells directly absorb these nanocrystals, which subsequently dissolve gradually in the cytoplasm to release active medication molecules. Both uptake and dissolution kinetics are influenced by variables like cell type, drug concentration, incubation duration, and polymeric surface coating (e.g., with Pluronic F68). Notably, surface coating increased cellular absorption and extended intracellular retention of the nanocrystals. Up to 50% of the internalized medication may stay in crystalline form, according to quantitative fluorescence and HPLC measurements, highlighting the need of intracellular dissolving for therapeutic efficacy. By employing environment-sensitive imaging agents, this method fills a significant knowledge gap regarding the dynamic behavior of medication nanocrystals after delivery and lays the groundwork for improving nanomedicine design [30]. The monodisperse $Gd_2O_3/Bi_2S_3$ nanodots created in this study are a logically designed class of multifunctional agents for cancer treatment that seamlessly combine imaging for diagnosis and treatment efficacy into a single nanosystem. Produced within a single albumin nanoreactor via simultaneous nanoprecipitation, these ultrasmall hybrid nanodots (~4.5 nm) utilize the structural compatibility of orthorhombic $Bi_3S_3$ and cubic $Gd_2O_3$ to create a uniform, stable architecture with high biocompatibility. They perform exceptionally well in multimodal imaging, providing superior CT imaging because of high X-ray attenuation of Bi, enhanced PA contrast from photothermal effects, and strong MR signals due to boosted longitudinal relaxivity. Under near-infrared irradiation, these nanodots exhibit a high photothermal conversion rate (~40%), strong photostability, and substantial tumor accumulation by clathrin-mediated endocytosis, which results in total tumor ablation with little damage. Excellent in vivo clearance and biodegradability are guaranteed by their albumin-based production, and imaging contrast may be optimized thanks to the adjustable Gd/Bi ratio. All things considered, these hybrid nanocrystals provide a potent and therapeutically applicable platform for non-invasive photothermal cancer treatment, real-time imaging, and accurate tumor localization [31].

## References

1. Chen, Y., Yan, C., Dong, J., Zhou, W., Rosei, F., Feng, Y., et al. (2021). Structure/property control in photocatalytic organic semiconductor nanocrystals. *Advanced Functional Materials, 31*(36), 2104099.
2. Kasai, H., Nakanishi, H., & Oikawa, H. (2018). Fabrication technique of organic nanocrystals and their optical properties and materialization. In *Nanoparticle Technology Handbook* (pp. 739–744): Elsevier.
3. Khan, S., Sharma, A., Ghoshal, S., Jain, S., Hazra, M. K., & Nandi, C. K. (2018). Small molecular organic nanocrystals resemble carbon nanodots in terms of their properties. *Chemical science, 9*(1), 175–180.
4. Marshall, C. R., Staudhammer, S. A., & Brozek, C. K. (2019). Size control over metal–organic framework porous nanocrystals. *Chemical science, 10*(41), 9396–9408.
5. Jrad, A., Damacet, P., Yaghi, Z., Ahmad, M., & Hmadeh, M. (2022). Zr-based metal–organic framework nanocrystals for water remediation. *ACS Applied Nano Materials, 5*(8), 10795–10808.
6. Li, M., Sun, M.-J., Yang, J., Huo, D., Lv, J., Shi, D., et al. (2022). Triplet–triplet energy transfer inside the single organic nanocrystal revealed by microscopic time resolved spectroscopy. *The Journal of Physical Chemistry C, 126*(27), 11033–11041.
7. Yang, Y., Wang, Y., Bai, F.-Q., Li, S.-X., Yang, Q., Wang, W., et al. (2024). Regulating planarized intramolecular charge transfer for efficient single-phase white-light emission in undoped metal–organic framework nanocrystals. *Nano Letters, 24*(32), 9898–9905.
8. Lu, D., Li, M., Gao, X., Yu, X., Wei, L., Zhu, S., et al. (2022). Cellulose nanocrystal films with NIR-II circularly polarized light for cancer detection applications. *ACS nano, 17*(1), 461–471.
9. Liu, Q., Kim, Y. J., Im, G. B., Zhu, J., Wu, Y., Liu, Y., et al. (2021). Inorganic nanoparticles applied as functional therapeutics. *Advanced Functional Materials, 31*(12), 2008171.
10. Núñez, C., Estévez, S. V., & del Pilar Chantada, M. (2018). Inorganic nanoparticles in diagnosis and treatment of breast cancer. *JBIC Journal of Biological Inorganic Chemistry, 23*, 331–345.
11. Wang, X., Zhong, X., Li, J., Liu, Z., & Cheng, L. (2021). Inorganic nanomaterials with rapid clearance for biomedical applications. *Chemical Society Reviews, 50*(15), 8669–8742.
12. An, D., Fu, J., Zhang, B., Xie, N., Nie, G., Ågren, H., et al. (2021). NIR-II responsive inorganic 2D nanomaterials for cancer photothermal therapy: recent advances and future challenges. *Advanced Functional Materials, 31*(32), 2101625.
13. Pugazhendhi, A., Edison, T. N. J. I., Karuppusamy, I., & Kathirvel, B. (2018). Inorganic nanoparticles: a potential cancer therapy for human welfare. *International journal of pharmaceutics, 539*(1-2), 104–111.
14. Lee, H. P., & Gaharwar, A. K. (2020). Light-responsive inorganic biomaterials for biomedical applications. *Advanced science, 7*(17), 2000863.

15. Chan, K. K., Giovanni, D., He, H., Sum, T. C., & Yong, K.-T. (2021). Water-stable all-inorganic perovskite nanocrystals with nonlinear optical properties for targeted multiphoton bioimaging. *ACS Applied Nano Materials, 4*(9), 9022–9033.
16. Kataoka, T., Abe, S., & Tagaya, M. (2019). Surface-engineered design of efficient luminescent europium (III) complex-based hydroxyapatite nanocrystals for rapid HeLa cancer cell imaging. *ACS Applied Materials & Interfaces, 11*(9), 8915–8927.
17. Pramanik, A., Patibandla, S., Gao, Y., Gates, K., & Ray, P. C. (2020). Water triggered synthesis of highly stable and biocompatible 1D nanowire, 2D nanoplatelet, and 3D nanocube CsPbBr3 perovskites for multicolor two-photon cell imaging. *JACS Au, 1*(1), 53–65.
18. Shen, W., Hu, T., Liu, X., Zha, J., Meng, F., Wu, Z., et al. (2022). Defect engineering of layered double hydroxide nanosheets as inorganic photosensitizers for NIR-III photodynamic cancer therapy. *Nature Communications, 13*(1), 3384.
19. Liu, Y., Zhang, G., Guo, Q., Ma, L., Jia, Q., Liu, L., et al. (2017). Artificially controlled degradable inorganic nanomaterial for cancer theranostics. *Biomaterials, 112*, 204–217.
20. Joseph, E., & Singhvi, G. (2019). Multifunctional nanocrystals for cancer therapy: a potential nanocarrier. *Nanomaterials for drug delivery and therapy*, 91–116.
21. Alejo, T., Sebastian, V., Mendoza, G., & Arruebo, M. (2022). Hybrid thermoresponsive nanoparticles containing drug nanocrystals for NIR-triggered remote release. *Journal of Colloid and Interface Science, 607*, 1466–1477.
22. Peng, J., Dong, M., Ran, B., Li, W., Hao, Y., Yang, Q., et al. (2017). "One-for-all"-type, biodegradable prussian blue/manganese dioxide hybrid nanocrystal for trimodal imaging-guided photothermal therapy and oxygen regulation of breast cancer. *ACS Applied Materials & Interfaces, 9*(16), 13875–13886.
23. Shen, X., Li, T., Chen, Z., Geng, Y., Xie, X., Li, S., et al. (2017). Luminescent/magnetic PLGA-based hybrid nanocomposites: a smart nanocarrier system for targeted codelivery and dual-modality imaging in cancer theranostics. *International journal of nanomedicine*, 4299–4322.
24. Debnath, T., Sarker, D., Huang, H., Han, Z.-K., Dey, A., Polavarapu, L., et al. (2021). Coherent vibrational dynamics reveals lattice anharmonicity in organic–inorganic halide perovskite nanocrystals. *Nature Communications, 12*(1), 2629.
25. Wang, Z., Li, J., Tu, W., Wang, H., Wang, Z., & Dai, Z. (2020). Formation of a photoelectrochemical Z-scheme structure with inorganic/organic hybrid materials for evaluation of receptor protein expression on the membrane of cancer cells. *ACS Applied Materials & Interfaces, 12*(24), 26905–26913.
26. Zhang, X., Yu, Y., Shen, J., Qi, W., & Wang, H. (2020). Design of organic/inorganic nanocomposites for ultrasensitive electrochemical detection of a cancer biomarker protein. *Talanta, 212*, 120794.
27. Muhammad, N., Zhao, H., Song, W., Gu, M., Li, Q., Liu, Y., et al. (2020). Silver nanoparticles functionalized Paclitaxel nanocrystals enhance overall anti-cancer effect on human cancer cells. *Nanotechnology, 32*(8), 085105.
28. Zhan, H., Zhou, X., Cao, Y., Jagtiani, T., Chang, T.-L., & Liang, J. F. (2017). Anti-cancer activity of camptothecin nanocrystals decorated by silver nanoparticles. *Journal of Materials Chemistry B, 5*(14), 2692–2701.
29. Mei, D., Gong, L., Zou, Y., Yang, D., Liu, H., Liang, Y., et al. (2020). Platelet membrane-cloaked paclitaxel-nanocrystals augment postoperative chemotherapeutical efficacy. *Journal of Controlled Release, 324*, 341–353.

30. Gao, W., Lee, D., Meng, Z., & Li, T. (2017). Exploring intracellular fate of drug nanocrystals with crystal-integrated and environment-sensitive fluorophores. *Journal of Controlled Release, 267*, 214–222.
31. Lv, X., Wang, X., Li, T., Wei, C., Tang, Y. a., Yang, T., et al. (2018). Rationally designed monodisperse Gd2O3/Bi2S3 hybrid nanodots for efficient cancer theranostics. *Small, 14*(49), 1802904.

# Nanocrystals Applications in Cancer Therapy 3

## 3.1 Introduction

Cancer persists as one of the top causes of morbidity and fatality across the globe, with an approximate 20 million new cases and 10 million deaths declared worldwide in 2023 alone [1]. Despite significant progress in quick diagnosis and medical care, the efficacy of standard cancer therapies such as chemotherapy, radiation, and immunotherapy is often restricted by several pharmacological and physiological challenges [2]. These include the limited solubility in water of many chemotherapeutic medicines, non-specific biodistribution, systemic toxicity, multidrug resistance, and heterogeneous tumor microenvironments [3]. As a result, there is an immediate need to promote novel platforms that can enhance the beneficial effects of drugs, improve tumor targeting, and minimize adverse effects [4].

Nanotechnology has arisen as a robust interdisciplinary method to addressing these restrictions by enabling the rational design of nanoscale drug delivery schemes that augment the pharmacokinetic and pharmacodynamic outlines of anticancer agents [5–7]. Among the various nanocarrier systems explored to date, including liposomes, dendrimers, polymeric nanoparticles, and micelles, nanocrystals embody a unique and highly adaptable class of drug delivery arrangements, especially well-suited for low water-soluble compounds [8–11].

Nanocrystals remain pure crystalline particles of a drug substance, stabilized by minimal amounts of surfactants or polymeric excipients [12, 13]. Unlike conventional nanoparticle systems, which encapsulate or conjugate the drug within a carrier matrix, nanocrystals consist almost entirely of the active pharmaceutical ingredient (API) [14, 15]. This high drug-loading capability translates to improved therapeutic payload per unit mass, reduced excipient toxicity, and efficient cellular uptake [11, 15, 16]. The enhanced surface area of nanocrystals leads to a substantial upsurge in dissolution rate, making them particularly effective for drugs characterized by poor water solubility but high permeability [17].

Nanocrystals have demonstrated significant promise as drug delivery vehicles in oncology, with the ability to be directed via numerous routes, comprising oral, intravenous, and pulmonary, depending on their morphology, size, and surface chemistry [18, 19]. When administered intravenously, nanocrystals can utilize the enhanced permeability and retention (EPR) effect to passively localize in tumor sites, taking advantage of dripping vasculature and diminished lymphatic drainage [20]. Furthermore, surface modification of nanocrystals with targeting moieties, including antibodies, peptides, or aptamers, can ease active targeting of tumor cells, thereby enabling selective uptake via receptor-mediated endocytosis and plummeting collateral toxicity to healthy cells [21–23].

The resulting formulations exhibited favorable physicochemical characteristics, including uniform spherical morphology, nanoscale size, and good physical stability [25]. Notably, the surface-modified $As_2O_3$@LA/PEG-PLGA nanoparticles displayed a controlled, moderate drug release profile. They presented enhanced cellular internalization and the highest cytotoxicity against the SMMC-7721 liver tumor cell line in vitro [25]. In vivo studies further confirmed that PEG/LA surface modification improved biocompatibility and reduced the general side effects typically associated with free $As_2O_3$ management. These findings support LA/PEG-PLGA nanoparticles as a promising and efficient nanoscale delivery technique for liver cancer cure [25].

In addition to functioning as delivery systems, specific nanocrystals themselves can exhibit intrinsic anticancer activity [26, 27]. For instance, nanocrystals composed of arsenic trioxide, curcumin, or camptothecin have demonstrated cytotoxic effects through innumerable mechanisms, including the orientation of oxidative stress, mitochondrial disruption, and interference with oncogenic signaling pathways [24, 28, 29]. For example, as shown in Fig. 3.1, research has demonstrated that surface-modified PLGA nanoformulations can significantly boost the therapeutic performance of arsenic trioxide ($As_2O_3$) for liver cancer therapy [24]. In a study by Song et al., $As_2O_3$-loaded PLGA nanoparticles were engineered using a dual emulsion-solvent evaporation method, supported by surface modification with polyethylene glycol (PEG) and/or lactic acid (LA) via covalent coupling [25]. FTIR analysis confirmed successful conjugation of PEG and LA onto the nanoparticle surface. lactic acid (LA) via covalent coupling [25]. FTIR analysis confirmed successful conjugation of PEG and LA onto the nanoparticle surface.

Furthermore, metal-based nanocrystals (e.g., gold, silver, selenium) have been shown to possess direct antitumor properties. They can also be utilized in blend with photothermal or photodynamic cure for enhanced efficacy [30]. The fabrication of nanocrystals involves either top-down approaches, such as high-pressure homogenization and wet milling, as well as bottom-up approaches, including antisolvent precipitation-controlled crystallization, each with its advantages and constraints of size control, scalability, and stability [31]. Recent advances in hybrid technologies, such as media milling followed by spray

## 3.1 Introduction

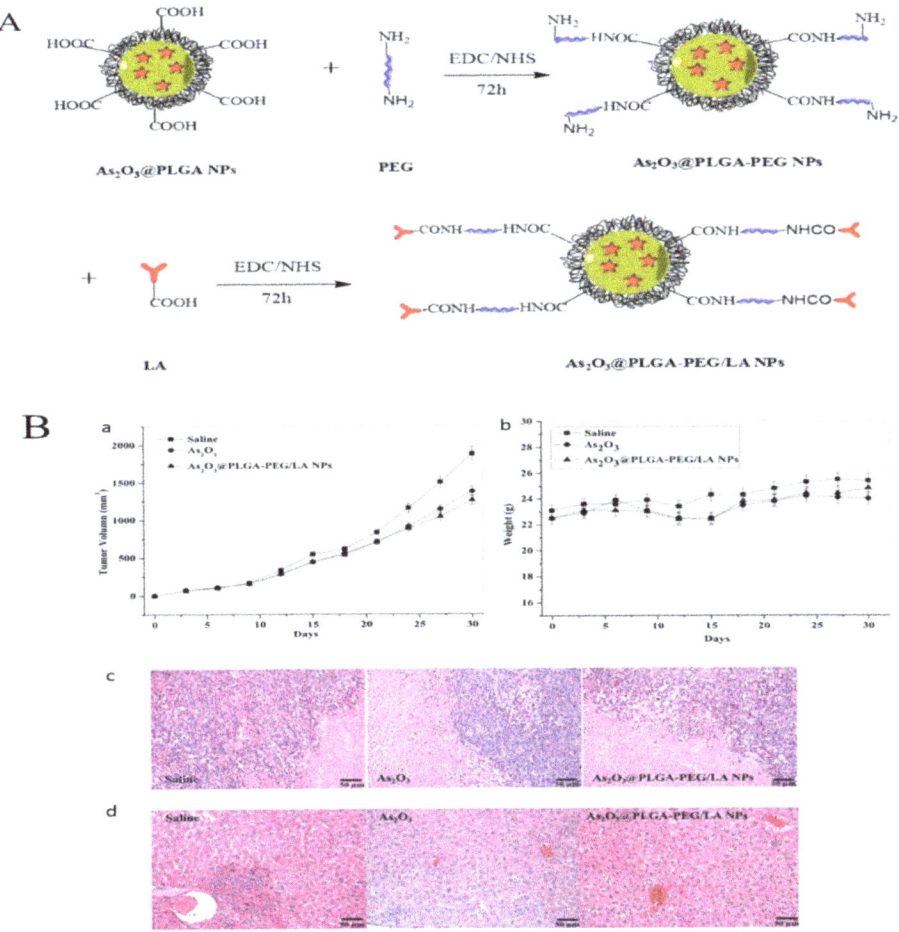

**Fig. 3.1** Surface modification and therapeutic evaluation of $As_2O_3$@PLGA nanoparticles. **a** Tumor growth curves in mice following intravenous administration of saline, free $As_2O_3$, or $As_2O_3$@PLGA-PEG/LA nanoparticles, demonstrating enhanced tumor suppression by the surface-modified formulation. **b** Monitoring body weight over time after injection indicates systemic tolerance to the treatment. **c** Symbolic H&E-stained liver portions, indicating histological changes and potential toxicity. **d** H&E-stained tumor sections, highlighting morphological differences and treatment efficacy across groups. Reused from the publication Ref. [24]

drying or lyophilization, have further improved the physical stability and processability of nanocrystal formulations [11, 31].

In spite of their immense conceivable, the medical translation of nanocrystals faces own challenges, including scale-up difficulties, long-term stability, regulatory complexities, and the need for vigorous in vivo reproductions to assess pharmacological behavior and safety [14, 32]. However, several nanocrystal-based formulations, such as Abraxane (nanoparticle albumin-bound paclitaxel), have already established FDA agreement, underscoring the feasibility of this approach in clinical oncology [33, 34].

This chapter delivers a wide-ranging examination of nanocrystals in the context of cancer therapy, structured into three key domains: (1) their application as drug delivery vehicles to enhance bioavailability and pharmacokinetics; (2) their role in targeted therapy through active and passive targeting mechanisms; and (3) their potential as direct anticancer agents through intrinsic cytotoxicity or as components in combination modalities. Emphasis is placed on mechanistic insights, formulation strategies, preclinical and clinical progress, and the translational considerations that will guide the future development of nanocrystal-based cancer therapeutics.

Standard nanocrystal-based drug delivery systems include.

## 3.2 Types of Nanocrystals

Nanocrystals are nanoscale crystalline particles (typically < 500 nm) with unique physicochemical assets that make them valuable in drug delivery and tumor therapy [35]. Based on composition and function, they can be classified into several types.

### 3.2.1 Organic Nanocrystals

Drug nanocrystals are pure, nanosized crystalline forms of active pharmaceutical ingredients (APIs), characteristically vacillating from 10 to 500 nm in size [13, 36]. These are composed entirely of the drug compound with no carrier matrix and display an elevated surface area-to-volume percentage, which enhances the suspension rate. Further, these do not require encapsulation or chemical alteration of the drug. Sometimes, these nanocrystals are stabilized using surfactants or polymers to prevent agglomeration and maintain a stable colloidal suspension [37]. Due to their tiny size and huge surface area, drug nanocrystals rapidly dissolve in physiological fluids, overcoming solubility-limited absorption. This allows for higher plasma concentrations and improved therapeutic efficacy of drugs with poor water solubility. For example, Paclitaxel, a potent chemotherapeutic agent with poor solubility in water, has been formulated as nanocrystals, such as Nanoxel or Abraxane; however, the latter is albumin-bound, allowing for intravenous administration without the need for toxic solvents like Cremophor EL [38, 39]. This improves patient safety, reduces hypersensitivity reactions, and enhances drug exposure at tumor sites [40].

## 3.2.2 Inorganic Nanocrystals

Inorganic nanocrystals are nanoscale particles made from non-carbon-based ingredients such as metal oxides, metals, or silica. Owing to their distinct physical, visual, magnetic, and chemical chattels, these nanocrystals have gained momentous attention in tumor diagnosis, imaging, and treatment [41]. For example, inorganic nanocrystals present the rational strategy and multifunctionality of a multimodal theranostic nanoparticle system for targeted tumor therapy and real-time imaging (as shown in Fig. 3.2) [42]. As illustrated in panel (a), the core consists of GZCIS ($Gd^{3+}$, $Zn^{2+}$, $Cu^+$, $In^{3+}$, $S^{2-}$) quantum dots (QDs), which are coated with a ZnS shell to enhance photostability and biocompatibility. These QDs are embedded into mesoporous silica nanoparticles (MSNs) using a CTAB-assisted microemulsion method, followed by surface silanization. The system is engineered for therapeutic efficacy through the loading of epirubicin (EPI) and functionalization with gold nanoparticles (Au NPs) for radiosensitization. Subsequent PEGylation improves colloidal stability and prolongs circulation time, while EpCAM-targeting aptamers are conjugated to facilitate tumor-specific active targeting [42]. Panel (b) summarizes the integrated therapeutic and diagnostic functions of the final construct (~65 nm in diameter), which enables: (1) active tumor targeting via aptamer-mediated recognition, (2) pH-responsive EPI release in acidic endosomal compartments, (3) radiotherapy enhancement via Au NPs, (4) improved systemic pharmacokinetics through PEGylation, and multimodal imaging through (5) CT (gold), (6) MRI (Gd), and (7) fluorescence (QDs). This innovative nanoparticle platform exemplifies a synergistic strategy for precision oncology, combining targeted drug delivery, enhanced therapeutic response, and real-time image-guided monitoring [42].

## 3.2.3 Hybrid Nanocrystals

Hybrid nanocrystals are advanced nanosystems that combine both organic and inorganic components within a single platform. This design synergizes the therapeutic adaptability of organic nanocarriers with the functional possessions of inorganic nanomaterials [43–45]. For example, a gold-polymer hybrid nanocrystal can deliver doxorubicin, provide imaging contrast, and generate heat for photothermal therapy all in one platform [46]. Each type offers unique rewards, such as improved stability, controlled drug release, targeted distribution, and imaging capabilities, making nanocrystals versatile tools in the field of nanomedicine. Next, we discuss key features and potential applications of different nano crystals. To start with, polymeric nanocrystals, such as individuals made from poly(lactic-co-glycolic acid) and PEGylated (polyethylene glycol-modified) systems, are at the forefront of controlled and prolonged drug release in cancer therapy [47]. These nanocrystals are engineered from biodegradable and biocompatible polymers,

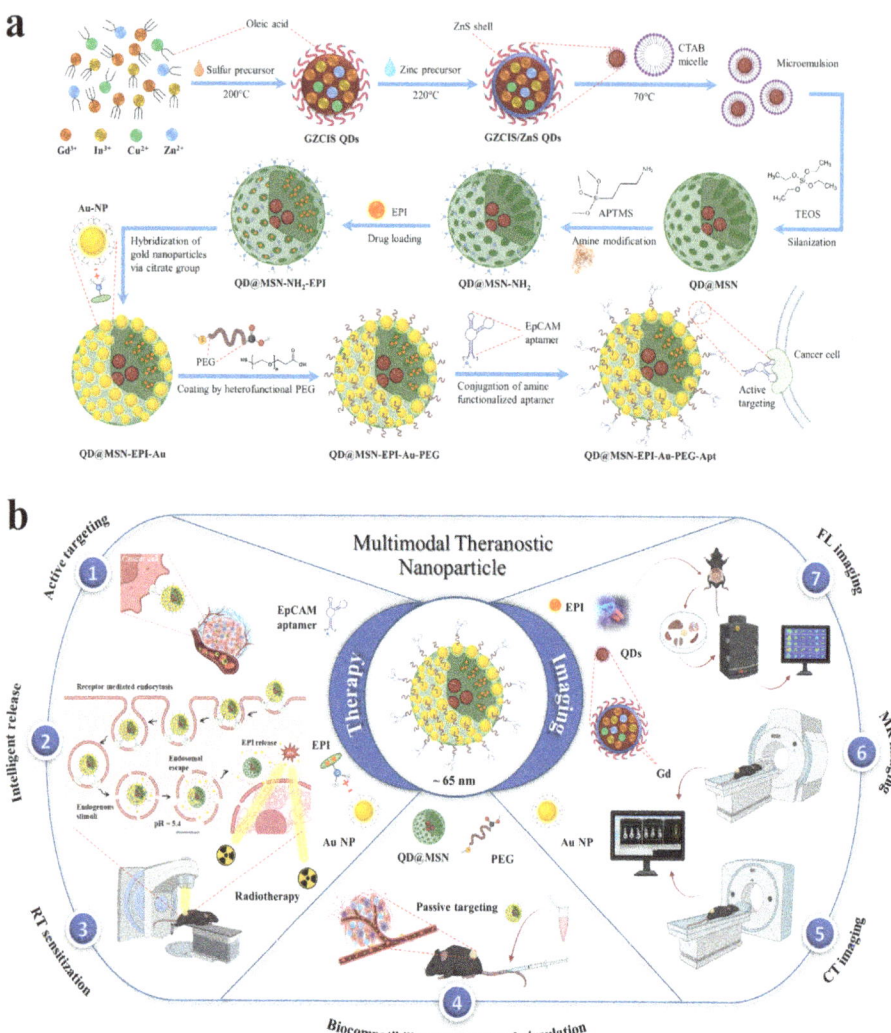

**Fig. 3.2** Design and multifunctional applications of the QD-MSN-EPI-Au-PEG@Apt nanoformulation. **a** Graphic representation of the stepwise groundwork of the theranostic nanocarrier, including the synthesis of quantum dots, encapsulation into mesoporous silica nanoparticles, surface modification with epirubicin (EPI), gold nanoparticles (Au NPs), polyethylene glycol (PEG), and EpCAM-targeting aptamers. **b** Overview of the multimodal capabilities of the final nanosystem for cancer theranostics, comprising targeted drug delivery, impetus-responsive release, radiosensitization, and multimodal imaging. Acronyms: QD, quantum dot; CTAB, $n$-cetyltrimethylammonium bromide; TEOS, tetraethyl orthosilicate; APTMS, (3-aminopropyl)trimethoxysilane; MSN, mesoporous silica nanoparticle; EPI, epirubicin; NP, nanoparticle; PEG, polyethylene glycol; EpCAM, epithelial cell adhesion molecule; RT, radiotherapy; CT, computed tomography; MR, magnetic resonance; FL, fluorescence. Figure adapted from the recent publication [42]

## 3.2 Types of Nanocrystals

which empower the encapsulation of a wide range of therapeutic agents, including small molecules, proteins, and nucleic acids [48].

**Key Features and Advantages of Polymeric Nanocrystals:**

- **Sustained and Controlled Release**: Polymeric nanocrystals can be persuaded to gradually release active agents over an extended period, ensuring consistent drug levels at the tumor spot while minimizing the need for recurrent dosing. This controlled release profile is achieved by fine-tuning the polymer composition, molecular weight, and nanocrystal morphology [49].
- **Enhanced Drug Stability and Bioavailability**: Encapsulating therapeutic agents within polymeric nanocrystal matrices provides a protective barrier against harsh physiological conditions, including enzymatic degradation, hydrolysis, and premature metabolism [50]. This protection significantly extends the drug's stability in systemic circulation. It enhances its bioavailability by ensuring that more of the active compound reaches the intended site of action in its functional form [51].
- **Targeted Distribution and Abbreviated Side Effects**: Surface functionalization with targeting ligands qualifies active targeting of tumor cells, increasing cellular uptake and minimalizing off-target effects [52]. PEGylation, especially, helps nanocrystals dodge the immune system and extend circulation time [52, 53].
- **Versatile Drug Loading**: The amphiphilic properties of many polymers permit for the competent encapsulation of both hydrophobic and hydrophilic drugs within a single nanocrystal platform. This versatility supports the codelivery of multiple therapeutic agents, making polymeric nanocrystals particularly well-suited for combination therapies targeting complex diseases such as cancer [54].
- **Overcoming Biological Barriers**: Polymeric nanocrystals can be deliberately designed to bypass endosomal entrapment by incorporating features that facilitate endosomal escape, including pH-subtle or membrane-disruptive components. This enables the direct release of therapeutic payloads into the cytoplasm, thereby improving intracellular delivery and significantly enhancing therapeutic efficacy [55].
- **Improved Patient Compliance**: Polymeric nanocrystal systems enable prolonged and sustained drug release, upholding therapeutic levels over prolonged periods. This reduces the need for regular dosing, simplifies treatment regimens, and ultimately enhances patient adherence, particularly in chronic or long-term therapies [56].

**Recent Advances**: Breakthroughs in nanofabrication techniques have enabled the expansion of polymeric nanocrystals with precisely tunable sizes, shapes, and surface characteristics. These advancements facilitate enhanced control over drug release profiles, biodistribution, and cellular uptake. Moreover, surface functionalization with targeting ligands has significantly improved the specificity and therapeutic efficacy of these nanocrystals in preclinical models of various cancers, including breast, ovarian, and colorectal malignancies. A recent paper illustrates the design, synthesis, and cellular application of a cationic cellulose nanocrystal (CNC)-based delivery system for polymeric siRNA in cancer therapy [57]. In the first step, native CNCs undergo hydrothermal desulfation to remove sulfate groups, followed by cationic surface modification using quaternary ammonium compounds, resulting in positively charged CNCs. These polymeric transcripts are released from the DNA scaffold via EDTA treatment, yielding structured polymeric siRNA strands. The cationic CNCs and negatively charged polymeric siRNA are then assembled into nanocomplexes via electrostatic interactions [57]. Upon administration, these nanocomplexes are taken up by cancer cells through endocytosis. Inside the cell, the polymeric siRNA is released, processed by the enzyme chopper, and incorporated into the RNA-induced silencing complex, leading to targeted gene silencing [57]. This approach highlights a promising non-viral strategy for siRNA delivery, offering enhanced stability, cellular uptake, and gene regulation for cancer therapeutics [57]. In summary, polymeric nanocrystals such as PLGA and PEGylated systems represent a highly adaptable and effective platform for controlled and prolonged drug release in cancer therapy, offering significant improvements in drug stability, targeting, and patient outcomes [58].

### 3.2.4 Lipid-Based Nanocrystals

Lipid-based nanocrystals, comprising liposomes and solid lipid nanoparticles, serve as highly efficient carriers for hydrophobic drugs, overcoming critical challenges related to poor aqueous solubility, limited bioavailability, and rapid degradation [59, 60]. These systems enhance drug stability, improve pharmacokinetic profiles, and enable targeted delivery, making them valuable tools in the formulation of effective and patient-friendly therapeutics [61].

**Key Features and Mechanisms**

- **Structure and Encapsulation**: Liposomes are spherical vesicles self-possessed of one or more phospholipid bilayers, offering a versatile architecture for drug encapsulation. Hydrophobic drugs are incorporated into the lipid bilayer, whereas hydrophilic drugs canister be enclosed within the aqueous central, enabling dual-loading capabilities [62]. In contrast, solid-lipid nanoparticles feature a solid lipid core alleviated by surfactants, which provides a robust matrix for the efficient entrapment of hydrophobic drugs. This solid core structure enhances drug stability, controls release kinetics and maintains nanoscale dimensions suitable for systemic delivery [63].
- **Enhanced Bioavailability**: The hydrophobic interior of lipid-based nanocrystals provides an ideal microenvironment for the solubilization of weekly water-soluble drugs [64]. By encapsulating these compounds, the systems protect them from premature degradation and facilitate their absorption across biological membranes. This results in significantly improved bioavailability, enhancing the overall therapeutic potential of the encapsulated drugs [64, 65].

## 3.2 Types of Nanocrystals

- **Controlled and Sustained Release**: The lipid coatings and core matrix of these nanocrystals canister be precisely persuaded to achieve precise and continuous drug release profiles [66]. For instance, incorporating pH-sensitive lipid components enables the nanoparticles to remain stable during circulation while triggering the selective release of drugs in the interior the acidic tumor microenvironment. This targeted release strategy not only prolongs systemic circulation time but also helps maintain effective therapeutic drug concentrations at the tumor location, improving therapy efficacy [67].
- **Biocompatibility and Safety**: These nanoparticles are inherently biocompatible and biodegradable due to their composition from naturally occurring lipids. This characteristic lessens the risk of toxicity and adverse effects often related with synthetic carriers, making them safer and more suitable for clinical applications [68].
- **Versatility in Drug Loading**: Lipid-based nanocrystals are capable of encapsulating a broad spectrum of hydrophobic drugs. Their structural properties can be tailored, such as by incorporating surfactants or blending with lipids to significantly enhance drug load capacity and retention, thereby improving formulation stability and therapeutic effectiveness [69].
- **Hybrid Structures**: Hybrid nanoformulations are advanced lipid-based nanocrystals that integrate both solid and liquid lipids within their core [70]. This hybrid lipid matrix introduces structural imperfections, which increase the capacity for drug entrapment and effectively minimize drug leakage. As a result, NLCs offer enhanced drug-lading efficiency and amended formulation steadiness compared to traditional formulations [71].
- **Morphology and Release Profiles**: The shape and size of lipid-based nanocrystals significantly influence their drug-loading capacity and release kinetics. For example, cubic or capsule-shaped carriers offer a larger surface area and increased porosity compared to spherical particles, which can enhance drug entrapment efficiency and enable more precise and precise drug release profiles personalized to therapeutic needs [72].
- **Stimuli-Responsive Release**: Lipid coatings can be engineered to respond to specific environmental triggers, such as the acidic pH found in tumor microenvironments. This design enables the nanocrystals to release their therapeutic payload preferentially at the target site, maximizing drug efficacy while minimizing premature release and systemic side effects during circulation [73].

Table 3.1 below highlights the structural differences, drug encapsulation strategies, and key advantages of three major lipid-based nanocarrier systems. It also includes their typical particle size ranges, clinical development status, and representative therapeutic applications. Liposomes feature phospholipid bilayers, allowing dual drug loading, with several FDA-approved formulations. SLNs offer high physical stability and controlled release, while NLCs, with their hybrid lipid core, provide improved drug loading and condensed leakage, making them promising platforms for next-generation drug delivery systems.

The Table 3.2 summarizes and contrasts the key features of lipid-based nanocrystals, such as liposomes, nanostructured lipid carriers, and solid lipid nanoparticles with polymeric nanocrystals, including poly (lactic-co-glycolic acid) and PEGylated systems. Parameters compared include drug loading efficiency, release profiles, bioavailability, biocompatibility, stability, targeting ability, immune response, manufacturing scalability, and clinical translation status. Lipid-based nanocrystals offer superior biocompatibility, versatility in drug encapsulation, and rapid cellular uptake, making them suitable for topical and mucosal delivery. Polymeric nanocrystals offer enhanced stability, controlled and prolonged release, and tunable surface properties, making them ideal for targeted systemic therapies. This comprehensive overview facilitates the selection of the most suitable nanocarrier platform based on therapeutic objectives and the characteristics of the drug.

**Summary of Comparative Efficiency**: Lipid-based nanocrystals excel at loading drugs, improving bioavailability and enabling controlled release, particularly for topical and mucosal delivery with low immunogenicity. Polymeric nanocrystals (PLGA, PEGylated) offer prolonged, controlled release and drug protection, making them suitable for long-term systemic therapies; however, they may have lower drug loading and potential immune risks. Hybrid lipid-polymer systems combine the strengths of both, providing improved drug distribution. The choice be contingent on drug chattels, release needs, administration route, and therapeutic goals.

## 3.3 Inorganic Nanocrystals

Inorganic nanocrystals, including gold nanoparticles (AuNPs) and iron oxide nanoparticles, have gained significant attention in cancer therapy due to their inimitable physicochemical possessions and multifunctional capabilities [8, 74]. These nanocrystals assist not only as carriers for targeted drug transfer but also as disparity agents for advanced tomography procedures such as magnetic resonance imaging, computed tomography, and photoacoustic imaging [74]. Their intrinsic optical, magnetic, and electronic characteristics enable simultaneous therapeutic and diagnostic functions often referred to as theranostics. Additionally, inorganic nanocrystals can indeed be engineered in terms of shape, size, surface chemistry, and functionalization with targeting ligands or therapeutic molecules [75]. This level of customization enhances their capability to selectively collect in tumor tissues via passive or active targeting mechanisms, thereby increasing therapeutic efficacy while minimizing toxicity. Moreover, some inorganic nanocrystals possess inherent therapeutic effects; for example, gold nanoparticles can alter near-infrared light to generate heat for photothermal therapy, and iron oxide nanoparticles can generate reactive oxygen species for magnetic hyperthermia [76]. Collectively, these attributes make

## 3.3 Inorganic Nanocrystals

**Table 3.1** Structural differences, drug encapsulation strategies, and key advantages of three major lipid-based nanocarrier systems

| Lipid-based nanocrystal type | Structure | Hydrophobic drug encapsulation | Key advantages | Particle size range nm | Clinical status | Example applications |
|---|---|---|---|---|---|---|
| Liposomes | One or more concentric phospholipid bilayers adjacent an aqueous core | Incorporated in the lipid bilayer, hydrophilic drugs in the aqueous core | Biocompatible, dual drug loading, customizable surface, controlled and stimuli-responsive release | 50–200 | Several FDA-approved products | Doxil®, AmBisome® |
| Solid lipid nanoparticles (SLNs) | Solid lipid matrix stabilized by surfactants | Entrapped within the solid lipid core | High stabili, sustained release, low toxicity, scalable | 50–1000 | Preclinical to clinical trials | Delivery of anticancer agents, anti-inflammatory drugs, topical formulations |
| Nanostructured lipid carriers (NLCs) | Hybrid solid/liquid lipid core with structural imperfections | Disordered hybrid core allows enhanced loading of hydrophobic drugs | Enhanced drug loading, reduced leakage, improved storage stability and circulation time | 50–500 | Preclinical to early clinical studies | Cancer therapy, dermal delivery, oral formulations for poorly soluble drugs |

**Table 3.2** Summarizes and contrasts the key features of lipid-based nanocrystals

| Feature | Lipid-based nanocrystals | Polymeric nanocrystals |
|---|---|---|
| Drug loading efficiency | High for hydrophobic drugs (SLNs, NLCs); liposomes can condense both hydrophobic and hydrophilic drugs | Generally lower, especially for hydrophobic drugs, unless using polymer–lipid hybrids or surface engineering |
| Release profile | Controlled or stimuli-responsive release (e.g., pH, temperature); NLCs reduce burst release | Precisely controlled and prolonged release driven by polymer degradation kinetics (e.g., hydrolysis) |
| Bioavailability | Enhanced solubility and membrane permeability improve absorption, particularly for BCS Class II and IV drugs | Improved via protection from degradation; may be slower to release, limiting rapid onset |
| Biocompatibility | Excellent; composed of physiological lipids. PEGylation enhances stealth properties | Biodegradable and generally safe, though some synthetic or high MW polymers may induce immune responses |
| Stability (physical/chemical) | NLCs and SLNs have enhanced physical stability over liposomes; liposomes are prone to fusion/leakage | High structural integrity and chemical solidity, ideal for long-term storage and complex formulations |
| Targeting capability | Easily functionalized with targeting ligands, effective in passive and active targeting | High potential for ligand attachment, multifunctional systems, and responsive delivery (pH, ROS, enzymes) |
| Systemic circulation time | Improved with PEGylation, NLCs, and SLNs may offer better retention than unmodified liposomes | PEGylation, stealth coatings, and charge modulation prolong circulation and slow clearance by the reticuloendothelial system (RES) |
| Cellular uptake | Rapid uptake via endocytosis; fusogenic lipids can promote membrane fusion and cytoplasmic release | Endocytosis-dependent uptake; release is limited by endosomal escape efficiency unless modified |
| Immune response | Low immunogenicity: Some immune recognition may be possible with repeated dosing, which is minimized by the use of PEG | Higher immunogenic risk if not well-optimized; surface modifications can be mitigated |

(continued)

## 3.3 Inorganic Nanocrystals

**Table 3.2** (continued)

| Feature | Lipid-based nanocrystals | Polymeric nanocrystals |
|---|---|---|
| Manufacturing scalability | Scalable via methods like high-pressure homogenization, extrusion, or thin-film hydration | Scalable using nanoprecipitation, emulsion-solvent evaporation, spray drying, etc |
| Shelf-life and storage | Liposomes are less stable unless lyophilized or stored in optimized conditions; SLNs/NLCs are more stable | Excellent shelf life; the polymer matrix protects the drug cargo from oxidation or hydrolysis |
| Surface modification | Surface functionalization is possible using polyethylene glycol (PEG), ligands, or polymers for targeting and stealth applications | Highly tunable surfaces for targeting, responsiveness, or codelivery (e.g., with imaging agents) |
| Toxicity profile | Generally low; lipid components are metabolized naturally. SLNs/NLCs offer safer alternatives to synthetic carriers | Depending on polymer type, degradation rate, and by-products, PLGA and PEG are well-tolerated |
| Cost of production | Relatively cost-effective; lipids are inexpensive, but process optimization is required for scale-up | It may involve higher synthesis costs for some polymers and more complex fabrication protocols |
| Environmental sensitivity | Sensitive to temperature, oxidation, and hydrolysis (especially liposomes) | Less sensitive to environmental stress; suitable for harsh processing or storage conditions |
| Codelivery capability | Effective for co-encapsulating hydrophilic and hydrophobic drugs or drug-gene combinations | Excellent for multidrug or drug–isRNA, drug-protein systems through polymer architecture control |
| Clinical translation | Several FDA/EMA-approved formulations (e.g., Doxil®, AmBisome®, Onivyde®); strong track record | Growing interest, some in clinical trials; slower regulatory progress due to complexity |

inorganic nanocrystals powerful platforms for integrated cancer diagnosis and treatment [76].

Additionally, Inorganic nanocrystals can be functionalized with a targeting agent to permit site-specific delivery of cytotoxic drugs. This targeted approach curtails systemic toxicity and lessens adverse effects on healthy tissues [77]. For instance, gold nanoparticles conjugated with anti-EGFR antibodies have been used to deliver gemcitabine directly to pancreatic tumors, demonstrating significant inhibition of tumor growth [78].

Further, Inorganic nanocrystals are widely utilized as versatile contrast agents across multiple imaging modalities, enabling enhanced tumor detection, real-time checking of drug delivery, and improved diagnostic accuracy.

- **Iron Oxide Nanoparticles (IONPs)**: These nanoparticles exhibit superparamagnetic properties, which make them extremely operative contrast agents for magnetic resonance imaging [79]. By altering the local magnetic field, IONPs enhance the MRI signal, allowing for accurate tumor site and real-time tracking of therapeutic agents within the body. Their biocompatibility and aptitude to be functionalized with targeting agents further improve imaging specificity and therapeutic monitoring [80].
- **Gold Nanoparticles (AuNPs) and Quantum Dots (QDs)**: Both AuNPs and QDs possess strong optical absorption and fluorescence properties. Gold nanoparticles are excellent for photoacoustic imaging due to their capacity to absorb near-infrared light and generate ultrasound signals [81]. Quantum dots, with size-changeable fluorescence emission and excellent brightness, serve as powerful tools for fluorescence imaging, providing high-resolution picturing of tumor cells and genetic procedures at the molecular level [82].
- **Gadolinium and Lanthanide-Created Nanoparticles**: These nanoparticles are extensively exploited as MRI contrast vehicles owing to their strong paramagnetic effects [83]. Gadolinium-based nanocrystals, in particular, enhance signal contrast by shortening the relaxation times of neighboring hydrogen photons [84]. Moreover, their surfaces can be engineered through targeting moieties to assist precise imaging of tumor tissues or disease markers, combining diagnostic precision with therapeutic potential.

By integrating these varied imaging capabilities, inorganic nanocrystals facilitate multimodal imaging approaches that combine anatomical, functional, and molecular information. This comprehensive imaging strategy improves the accurateness of cancer diagnosis, guides personalized treatment plans, and enables non-invasive examining of therapeutic response [85].

Furthermore, Inorganic nanocrystals play a paramount role in expanding theranostics, an innovative approach that opens up therapeutic and diagnostic functionalities into a single platform [77]. By uniting targeted drug transport with real-time imaging competencies, these nanocrystals enable clinicians to visualize the spreading and growth of therapeutic agents directly within the patient's body. This twin functionality allows for the precise localization of cancers, monitoring of drug release, and assessment of treatment response simultaneously [86]. For example, iron oxide nanoparticles cannister assist as MRI contrast mediators while carrying chemotherapeutic drugs, permitting for concurrent tumor imaging and therapy. Similarly, gold nanoparticles can be exploited for photothermal therapy and tracked via photoacoustic tomography, providing immediate feedback on the treatment's effectiveness. Such real-time monitoring enhances the ability

## 3.3 Inorganic Nanocrystals

to adjust dosing regimens dynamically, improving therapeutic results and tumbling side effects [87].

Moreover, theranostic nanocrystals ease personalized medicine by custom handling plans based on individual persistent imaging data and biological responses. This incorporation supports early detection of treatment resistance or disease progression, enabling timely intervention and optimization of therapy [88]. The multifunctional design of inorganic nanocrystals also enables the combination of numerous therapeutic modes, such as chemotherapy, photothermal therapy, and immunotherapy, inside a nanoplatform. Overall, inorganic nanocrystal-based theranostics represent a transformative strategy in oncology, bridging diagnostics and treatment to enhance precision, efficacy, and patient outcomes [89].

### 3.3.1 Photothermal and Photodynamic Therapy

Gold and other metal-based inorganic nanocrystals possess unique optical and electronic characteristics that enable them to assist as effective agents in photodynamic therapy and photothermal therapy, two acerbic-edge modalities for cancer treatment [90].

### 3.3.2 Photothermal Therapy (PTT)

Gold nanoparticles and similar metal nanocrystals efficiently engage near-infrared (NIR) light, a wavelength that penetrates tissues deeply with trifling damage to nearby healthy cells [91]. Upon exposure to NIR light, these nanoparticles translate the absorbed light energy into localized heat, thereby hovering the temperature in the tumor microenvironment and inducing cancer cell death through hyperthermia. This targeted thermal ablation causes protein denaturation and disrupts cellular membranes, resulting in the apoptosis or necrosis of tumor cells. PTT offers spatial precision, minimizing collateral damage to normal tissues [92].

### 3.3.3 Photodynamic Therapy (PDT)

Certain metal nanocrystals, when conjugated with photosensitizing agents, can generate reactive oxygen species, such as singlet oxygen, upon activation by specific wavelengths of light [93]. These ROS cause oxidative damage to tumor cells, which is important for cell death over apoptosis or mortification [94]. PDT is minimally invasive and can be repeated multiple times without significant systemic toxicity. Moreover, the localized generation of ROS spares surrounding healthy tissues and vasculature [94].

### 3.3.4 Combination with Drug Delivery

Integrating PTT and PDT with chemotherapeutic drug delivery enhances anticancer efficacy through synergistic mechanisms. Inorganic nanocrystals can simultaneously act as carriers for cytotoxic drugs while providing photothermal or photodynamic effects [95]. This multimodal approach enables lower drug doses, thereby reducing systemic toxicity, and overcomes drug resistance by targeting tumors through multiple pathways. Furthermore, the light-triggered release of medications from nanoparticles can be precisely meticulous both spatially and temporally, thereby optimizing therapeutic outcomes. Figure 3.3 illustrates the synergistic use of porphysome-enabled photodynamic therapy and photothermal therapy in tumor therapy, highlighting the advantages of combining these modalities through nanomedicine [96]. Panel A depicts the experimental workflow, where porphysome nanoparticles are engineered to serve as both photothermal and photodynamic agents, enabling heat generation for PTT and reactive oxygen species production for PDT upon light activation. Panel B presents MRI thermometry images demonstrating the localized temperature increase achieved during porphysome-mediated PTT, with significant thermal elevation observed in treated regions compared to controls. Panel C quantitatively tracks temperature changes over time, confirming the efficient and sustained photothermal effect of porphysome-PTT relative to laser-only controls. Panel D focuses on the therapeutic outcomes of porphysome-enabled PDT, demonstrating tumor growth inhibition and improved survival in treated groups, as evidenced by tumor images and survival curves over a 30-day period. Collectively, results underscores how the combination of PDT and PTT via multifunctional porphysome nanoparticles leverages their distinct mechanisms for enhanced cancer therapy, as discussed in the referenced ACS Nano publication on photodynamic and photothermal synergy in nanomedicine [96].

Collectively, photothermal and photodynamic therapies enabled by metal nanocrystals represent a promising strategy in cancer treatment, offering targeted, minimally invasive options with enhanced efficacy when combined with conventional therapies.

### 3.3.5 Magnetic Manipulation

Iron oxide nanocrystals demonstrate superparamagnetic assets, enabling them to be directed and concentrated at tumor locations utilizing externally applied magnetic fields [97]. This magnetic guidance improves the gathering of therapeutic agents, surrounded explicitly by the tumor microenvironment, significantly increasing neighborhood drug concentrations while curtailing systemic distribution and associated side effects. By applying an external magnetic field, clinicians can non-invasively steer iron oxide nanoparticles through the bloodstream to the target tissue, thereby improving targeting precision beyond passive accumulation mechanisms, such as the enhanced permeability and retention effect [98].

## 3.3 Inorganic Nanocrystals

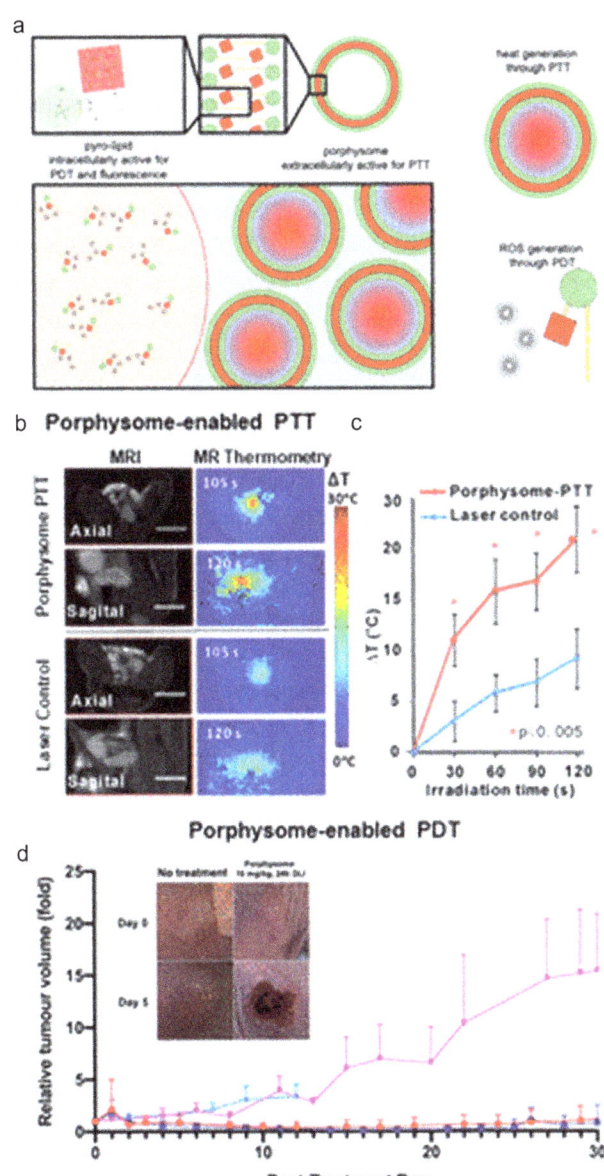

**Fig. 3.3** Porphysomes as twin PTT/PDT agents: **a** schematic showing porphysome structure and function. Intact porphysomes remain quenched but harvest heat upon 671 nm laser irradiation (PTT). Upon cellular uptake and disassembly, ROS generation is activated (PDT). **b** MR-thermometry in an orthotopic prostate tumor model showing significant temperature rise after porphysome injection and laser treatment. **c** Quantification of temperature increase during PTT (mean ± SD, n = 5). **d** Tumor volume changes in A549 tumor-bearing mice over 30 days following treatment with porphysome-PDT, photofrin-PDT, porphysomes alone, or photofrin alone (mean ± SD, n = 5). Adapted from a published ACS Nano journal [96]

Additionally, magnetic manipulation can be combined with magnetic resonance imaging to facilitate real-time tracking of nanoparticle biodistribution and deposition. This dual functionality facilitates personalized dosing and treatment adjustments based on imaging feedback [99]. The ability to spatially control nanoparticle delivery also opens avenues for magnetically triggered drug release, where alternating magnetic fields induce localized heating (magnetic hyperthermia) or mechanical effects that promote drug release from the nanoparticle carrier [100]. Overall, magnetic manipulation of iron oxide nanocrystals represents a powerful approach for ornamental the specificity, usefulness, and safety of cancer therapies through precise, externally controlled delivery [100].

In summary, inorganic nanocrystals, such as gold and iron oxide nanoparticles, provide a nifty podium that integrates targeted drug distribution with multiple imaging methods. Their surfaces can be tailored for selective targeting of cancer cells, and their release profiles can be engineered for controlled stimulus-responsive drug delivery. Additionally, these nanocrystals enable real-time tracking of drug distribution and treatment efficacy, positioning them as valuable tools for advancing precise, personalized, and minimally invasive cancer therapies [101]. From the above sections summarized in detail, nanocrystals significantly advance targeted cancer therapy by enabling the accurate delivery of therapeutic agents directly to tumor cells while lessening damage to healthy cells. Through surface functionalization with targeting agents, nanocrystals can explicitly bind to overexpressed receptors on cancer cells, thereby enhancing their uptake and efficacy. They can be engineered for stimuli-responsive drug release triggered by tumor-specific cues like pH or enzymes, ensuring localized action and reduced systemic toxicity.

Additionally, nanocrystals accelerate combination therapies by co-delivering several agents to overcome drug battle and improve outcomes. Their nanoscale size assists passive accumulation in tumors through the enhanced permeability and retention effect, while active targeting enhances discrimination. Nanocrystals improve drug stability and pharmacokinetics, offer high drug loading capacity for diverse molecules, and support controlled, sustained release to maintain therapeutic levels. By concentrating drugs at tumor sites, they reduce systemic side effects and cardiotoxicity, as demonstrated by PEGylated liposomal formulations. Moreover, nanocrystals can bypass resistance mechanisms and be administered through several routes. Overall, nanocrystal-based targeted therapies provide a versatile and practical platform for safer, more personalized cancer treatment.

## 3.4 Nanocrystals as Anticancer Agents

Beyond their role as drug delivery vehicles, specific nanocrystals exhibit intrinsic anticancer properties that can directly contribute to tumor eradication [77]. These multifunctional nanomaterials harness unique physical and chemical characteristics to induce cancer cell death through various mechanisms:

Photothermal and photodynamic agents competently recognize light energy and transfer it into heat or generate reactive oxygen species upon irradiation. In photothermal therapy, localized heating induces hyperthermia that selectively damages cancer cells while sparing adjacent healthy cells. Photodynamic therapy utilizes light-activated reactive oxygen species generation to persuade oxidative damage and apoptosis in tumor cells.

## 3.4 Nanocrystals as Anticancer Agents

The precise spatiotemporal control of light activation allows for minimally invasive treatment with reduced side effects. The recent liturature provides compelling in vivo evidence supporting the therapeutic potential of engineered HyNP3 quantum dot nanoparticles for photodynamic therapy in cancer treatment [102]. In a murine tumor model, administration of HyNP3 followed by light irradiation led to a marked reduction in tumor volume compared to all control groups, highlighting the enhanced therapeutic efficacy of the QD-based platform. Notably, body weight remained stable across all treatment conditions, suggesting that the nanoparticles exhibit favorable biocompatibility and low systemic toxicity [102]. Visual inspection of tumor tissues further confirmed these findings, with notably smaller tumors observed in the HyNP3 + light group. Histological analyses revealed a decrease in tumor cell density, as indicated by H&E staining, and an increase in apoptotic activity, as evidenced by strong TUNEL-positive fluorescence signals in the treated class [102]. These results collectively underscore the capability of rationally designed semiconductor QDs to generate reactive oxygen species, particularly singlet oxygen ($^1O_2$), and effectively mediate tumor suppression through targeted PDT. The study exemplifies how surface-engineered QDs can be leveraged as multifunctional nanotherapeutics in precision oncology [102].

### 3.4.1 Radiosensitizers

Nanocrystals composed of high atomic number elements improve the efficacy of radiotherapy by growing the deposition of ionizing radiation within tumor tissues [103]. These nanocrystals amplify the radiation dose locally, foremost to increased DNA impairment and cell death in cancer cells while diminishing introduction to surrounding normal tissues. This radiosensitizing effect improves therapeutic outcomes and may enable lower radiation doses, thereby reducing adverse effects [103, 104].

### 3.4.2 Direct Cytotoxicity

Certain inorganic nanocrystals, including quantum dots and metal oxide nanoparticles, can exert direct cytotoxic effects on cancer cells. Their unique surface chemistries facilitate interactions with cellular membranes and organelles, inducing oxidative stress, disrupting mitochondrial function, or triggering apoptotic pathways. These mechanisms contribute to tumor cell death independent of delivered drugs or external stimuli [105].

## 3.4.3 Combination Therapies

Nanocrystals can be engineered as versatile platforms to integrate multiple therapeutic modalities within a single construct [106]. By co-delivering chemotherapeutic agents alongside photothermal or immunotherapeutic components, these multifunctional systems maximize anticancer efficacy through synergistic mechanisms. Combining therapies also helps to overawed drug resistance, a significant challenge in cancer treatment, by simultaneously targeting multiple pathways involved in tumor survival and progression. Peng et al. developed a novel liposomal codelivery arrangement modified with HER-2 antibodies and mannose for the targeted treatment of lung cancer as shown in Fig. 3.4 [107]. This system simultaneously delivers vorinostat and gefitinib to modulate the tumor redox microenvironment and overcome drug resistance. Vorinostat, a histone deacetylase (HDAC) inhibitor, facilitated the repolarization of tumor-associated macrophages. Additionally, the liposomal formulation enhanced reactive oxygen species creation in cancer cells, thereby fluctuating the intracellular redox balance signaling pathway, ultimately resensitizing resistant cancer cells to gefitinib treatment [107].

In summary, nanocrystals represent a versatile and transformative platform in cancer therapy, offering both intrinsic anticancer properties and the capability to serve as erudite drug delivery schemes. Their unique physicochemical characteristics, including high surface area, tunable size, and customizable surface chemistry, enable precise drug loading, controlled release, and targeted delivery to tumor sites. Moreover, specific nanocrystals possess inherent therapeutic functions, including photothermal, photodynamic, and radiosensitizing effects, which allow them to directly induce tumor cell death or enhance the efficacy of conventional therapies. By participating in diagnostic and therapeutic functions, nanocrystals can also serve as theranostic agents, enabling the real-time monitoring of therapeutic responses. Importantly, their multifunctionality provides a strategic advantage in overcoming common challenges in oncology, such as multidrug resistance, off-target toxicity, and poor drug solubility. As research progresses, the rational design and clinical translation of nanocrystal-based platforms hold significant promise for advancing personalized and precision cancer treatments.

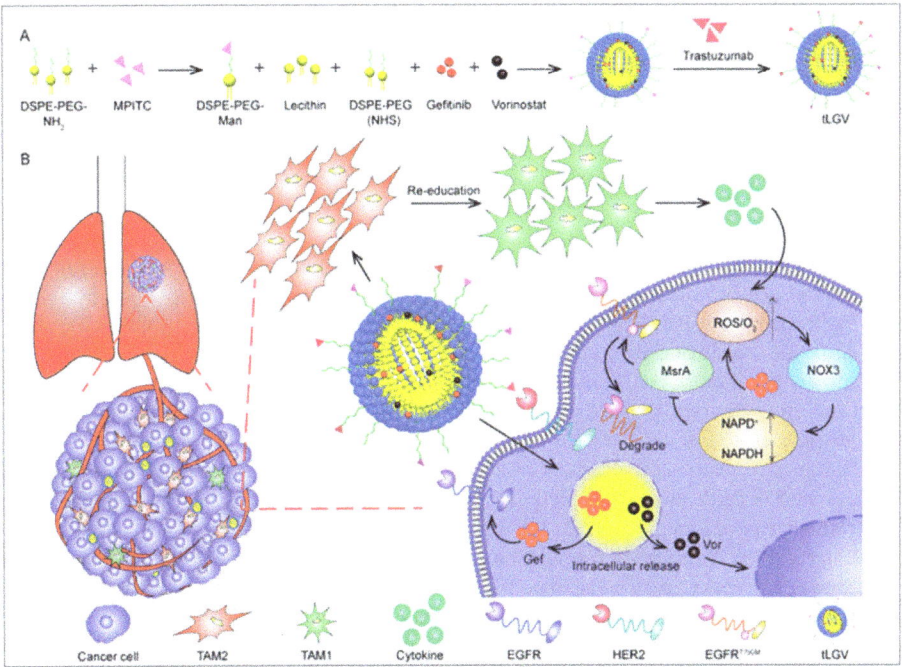

**Fig. 3.4** Schematic illustration of multifunctional nanocrystal-based combination therapy for targeted cancer treatment and tumor microenvironment modulation. **a** Schematic of tLGV nanocrystal assembly: DSPE-PEG derivatives are sequentially conjugated with MPITC, mannose, lectin, gefitinib, and vorinostat, then surface-functionalized with trastuzumab. **b** Mechanism of action: tLGV targets lung tumors, delivers gefitinib and vorinostat to cancer cells, increases ROS, disrupts redox balance, and reprograms TAM2 macrophages to TAM1, enhancing cytokine-mediated antitumor responses. Adapted from [107]

## References

1. Chhikara, B. S., & Parang, K. (2023). Global Cancer Statistics 2022: the trends projection analysis. *Chemical Biology Letters, 10*(1), 451.
2. Zafar, A., Khatoon, S., Khan, M. J., Abu, J., & Naeem, A. (2025). Advancements and limitations in traditional anti-cancer therapies: a comprehensive review of surgery, chemotherapy, radiation therapy, and hormonal therapy. *Discover Oncology, 16*(1), 607, https://doi.org/10.1007/s12672-025-02198-8.
3. Shao, X., Zhao, X., Wang, B., Fan, J., Wang, J., & An, H. (2025). Tumor microenvironment targeted nano-drug delivery systems for multidrug resistant tumor therapy. *Theranostics, 15*(5), 1689–1714, https://doi.org/10.7150/thno.103636.
4. Liu, G., Yang, L., Chen, G., Xu, F., Yang, F., Yu, H., et al. (2021). A review on drug delivery system for tumor therapy. *Frontiers in pharmacology, 12*, 735446.

5. Theivendren, P., Kunjiappan, S., Pavadai, P., Ravi, K., Murugavel, A., Dayalan, A., et al. (2024). Revolutionizing cancer immunotherapy: emerging nanotechnology-driven drug delivery systems for enhanced therapeutic efficacy. *ACS Measurement Science Au, 5*(1), 31–55.
6. Emeihe, E. V., Nwankwo, E. I., Ajegbile, M. D., Olaboye, J. A., & Maha, C. C. (2024). Revolutionizing drug delivery systems: Nanotechnology-based approaches for targeted therapy. *International Journal of Life Science Research Archive, 7*(1), 040–058.
7. Waje, M., & Balaiya, G. K. (2024). ADVANCEMENTS AND CHALLENGES IN DRUG DELIVERY SYSTEMS A COMPREHENSIVE REVIEW. *International Journal of Creative Research Thought*.
8. Yenurkar, D., Nayak, M., & Mukherjee, S. (2023). Recent advances of nanocrystals in cancer theranostics. *Nanoscale Advances, 5*(16), 4018–4040.
9. Mukherjee, S., & Pal, A. K. (2008). Size-dependent magnetic properties of VO2 nanocrystals dispersed in a silica matrix. *Journal of Physics: Condensed Matter, 20*(25), 255202.
10. Nayak, M., Kumar, V., Banerjee, D., Pradhan, L., Kamath, P., & Mukherjee, S. (2025). Quercetin nanocrystal-loaded alginate hydrogel patch for wound healing applications. *Journal of Materials Chemistry B, 13*(5), 1690–1703.
11. Pardhi, V. P., Verma, T., Flora, S., Chandasana, H., & Shukla, R. (2018). Nanocrystals: an overview of fabrication, characterization and therapeutic applications in drug delivery. *Current pharmaceutical design, 24*(43), 5129–5146.
12. Liu, P. (2013). Nanocrystal formulation for poorly soluble drugs. *University of Helsinki*, 1–70.
13. Dhaval, M., Makwana, J., Sakariya, E., & Dudhat, K. (2020). Drug nanocrystals: a comprehensive review with current regulatory guidelines. *Current drug delivery, 17*(6), 470–482.
14. Chary, P. S., Shaikh, S., Bhavana, V., Rajana, N., Vasave, R., & Mehra, N. K. (2024). Emerging role of nanocrystals in pharmaceutical applications: A review of regulatory aspects and drug development process. *Applied Materials Today, 40*, 102334.
15. Ding, Y., Zhao, T., Fang, J., Song, J., Dong, H., Liu, J., et al. (2024). Recent developments in the use of nanocrystals to improve bioavailability of APIs. *Wiley Interdisciplinary Reviews: Nanomedicine and Nanobiotechnology, 16*(2), e1958.
16. Kalhapure, R. S., Palekar, S., Patel, K., & Monpara, J. (2022). Nanocrystals for controlled delivery: state of the art and approved drug products. *Expert opinion on drug delivery, 19*(10), 1303–1316.
17. Liu, T., Yu, X., Yin, H., & Möschwitzer, J. P. (2019). Advanced modification of drug nanocrystals by using novel fabrication and downstream approaches for tailor-made drug delivery. *Drug delivery, 26*(1), 1092–1103.
18. Zingale, E., Bonaccorso, A., Carbone, C., Musumeci, T., & Pignatello, R. (2022). Drug nanocrystals: focus on brain delivery from therapeutic to diagnostic applications. *Pharmaceutics, 14*(4), 691.
19. Chen, W., Huang, J., Guo, Y., Wang, X., Lin, Z., Wei, R., et al. (2025). Nanocrystals for Intravenous Drug Delivery: Composition Development, Preparation Methods and Applications in Oncology. *AAPS PharmSciTech, 26*(3), 66.
20. Zi, Y., Yang, K., He, J., Wu, Z., Liu, J., & Zhang, W. (2022). Strategies to enhance drug delivery to solid tumors by harnessing the EPR effects and alternative targeting mechanisms. *Advanced Drug Delivery Reviews, 188*, 114449.
21. Kunjiappan, S., Pavadai, P., Vellaichamy, S., Ram Kumar Pandian, S., Ravishankar, V., Palanisamy, P., et al. (2021). Surface receptor-mediated targeted drug delivery systems for enhanced cancer treatment: A state-of-the-art review. *Drug Development Research, 82*(3), 309–340.
22. Anarjan, F. S. (2019). Active targeting drug delivery nanocarriers: Ligands. *Nano-Structures & Nano-Objects, 19*, 100370.

23. Karra, N., & Benita, S. (2012). The ligand nanoparticle conjugation approach for targeted cancer therapy. *Current drug metabolism, 13*(1), 22–41.
24. Yu, M., Zhang, Y., Fang, M., Jehan, S., & Zhou, W. (2022). Current Advances of Nanomedicines Delivering Arsenic Trioxide for Enhanced Tumor Therapy. *Pharmaceutics, 14*(4), 743.
25. Song, X., You, J., Shao, H., & Yan, C. (2018). Effects of surface modification of As(2)O(3)-loaded PLGA nanoparticles on its anti-liver cancer ability: An in vitro and in vivo study. *Colloids Surf B Biointerfaces, 169*, 289–297, https://doi.org/10.1016/j.colsurfb.2018.05.024.
26. Khairnar, P., Handa, M., & Shukla, R. (2022). Nanocrystals: an approachable delivery system for anticancer therapeutics. *Current drug metabolism, 23*(8), 603–615.
27. Pileni, M.-P. (2007). Self-assembly of inorganic nanocrystals: fabrication and collective intrinsic properties. *Accounts of chemical research, 40*(8), 685–693.
28. Wang, S., Liu, C., Wang, C., Ma, J., Xu, H., Guo, J., et al. (2020). Arsenic trioxide encapsulated liposomes prepared via copper acetate gradient loading method and its antitumor efficiency. *Asian J Pharm Sci, 15*(3), 365–373, https://doi.org/10.1016/j.ajps.2018.12.002.
29. Sarkar, N., Das, B., Bishayee, A., & Sinha, D. (2019). Arsenal of Phytochemicals to Combat Against Arsenic-Induced Mitochondrial Stress and Cancer. *Antioxidants & Redox Signaling, 33*(17), 1230–1256, https://doi.org/10.1089/ars.2019.7950.
30. Sun, Y., Li, Q., Huang, Y., Yang, Z., Li, G., Sun, X., et al. (2024). Natural products for enhancing the sensitivity or decreasing the adverse effects of anticancer drugs through regulating the redox balance. *Chinese Medicine, 19*(1), 110.
31. Mohana Raghava Srivalli, K., & Mishra, B. (2015). Drug nanocrystals: four basic prerequisites for formulation development and scale-up. *Current Drug Targets, 16*(2), 136–147.
32. Yadav, A., Thakur, P., Thakur, A., & Suhag, D. (2025). Challenges in Scaling Nanobiology for Clinical Use. In *Advancements in Nanobiology* (pp. 303–317): CRC Press.
33. Murphy, G., Brayden, D. J., Cheung, D. L., Liew, A., Fitzgerald, M., & Pandit, A. (2025). Albumin-based delivery systems: Recent advances, challenges, and opportunities. *Journal of Controlled Release, 380*, 375–395, https://doi.org/10.1016/j.jconrel.2025.01.035.
34. Samad, M. A., Ahmad, I., Zughaibi, T. A., Suhail, M., Zaidi, S. K., Al-Abbasi, F. A., et al. (2025). Nanotechnology-based drug delivery for breast cancer treatment: Current applications and future directions. *European Journal of Medicinal Chemistry Reports, 14*, 100268, https://doi.org/10.1016/j.ejmcr.2025.100268.
35. Pardhi, V. P., Verma, T., Flora, S. J. S., Chandasana, H., & Shukla, R. (2018). Nanocrystals: An Overview of Fabrication, Characterization and Therapeutic Applications in Drug Delivery. *Curr Pharm Des, 24*(43), 5129–5146, https://doi.org/10.2174/1381612825666190215121148.
36. Peltonen, L., Hirvonen, J., & Laaksonen, T. (2014). Drug nanocrystals and nanosuspensions in medicine. In *Handbook of nanobiomedical research: Fundamentals, applications and recent developments: Volume 1. Materials for nanomedicine* (pp. 169–197): World Scientific.
37. Tuomela, A., Hirvonen, J., & Peltonen, L. (2016). Stabilizing agents for drug nanocrystals: effect on bioavailability. *Pharmaceutics, 8*(2), 16.
38. Gradishar, W. J. (2006). Albumin-bound paclitaxel: a next-generation taxane. *Expert Opin Pharmacother, 7*(8), 1041–1053, https://doi.org/10.1517/14656566.7.8.1041.
39. Desai, N. (2016). Nanoparticle Albumin-Bound Paclitaxel (Abraxane®). In M. Otagiri, & V. T. G. Chuang (Eds.), *Albumin in Medicine: Pathological and Clinical Applications* (pp. 101–119). Singapore: Springer Singapore.
40. Cucinotto, I., Fiorillo, L., Gualtieri, S., Arbitrio, M., Ciliberto, D., Staropoli, N., et al. (2013). Nanoparticle albumin bound Paclitaxel in the treatment of human cancer: nanodelivery reaches prime-time? *J Drug Deliv, 2013*, 905091, https://doi.org/10.1155/2013/905091.

41. Wang, W., Zhang, M., Pan, Z., Biesold, G. M., Liang, S., Rao, H., et al. (2022). Colloidal Inorganic Ligand-Capped Nanocrystals: Fundamentals, Status, and Insights into Advanced Functional Nanodevices. *Chemical Reviews, 122*(3), 4091–4162, https://doi.org/10.1021/acs.chemrev.1c00478.
42. Abrishami, A., Bahrami, A. R., Nekooei, S., Sh. Saljooghi, A., & Matin, M. M. (2024). Hybridized quantum dot, silica, and gold nanoparticles for targeted chemo-radiotherapy in colorectal cancer theranostics. *Communications Biology, 7*(1), 393, https://doi.org/10.1038/s42003-024-06043-6.
43. Ananikov, V. P. (2019). Organic-Inorganic Hybrid Nanomaterials. *Nanomaterials (Basel), 9*(9), https://doi.org/10.3390/nano9091197.
44. Lu, Y., Lv, Y., & Li, T. (2019). Hybrid drug nanocrystals. *Advanced Drug Delivery Reviews, 143*, 115–133, https://doi.org/10.1016/j.addr.2019.06.006.
45. Bruckner, E. P., Curk, T., Đorđević, L., Wang, Z., Yang, Y., Qiu, R., et al. (2022). Hybrid Nanocrystals of Small Molecules and Chemically Disordered Polymers. *ACS Nano, 16*(6), 8993–9003, https://doi.org/10.1021/acsnano.2c00266.
46. Dong, Q., Wan, C., Yang, H., Zheng, D., Xu, L., Zhou, Z., et al. (2020). Targeted gold nanoshelled hybrid nanocapsules encapsulating doxorubicin for bimodal imaging and near-infrared triggered synergistic therapy of Her2-positve breast cancer. *J Biomater Appl, 35*(3), 430–445, https://doi.org/10.1177/0885328220929616.
47. Zhang, D., Liu, L., Wang, J., Zhang, H., Zhang, Z., Xing, G., et al. (2022). Drug-loaded PEG-PLGA nanoparticles for cancer treatment. *Front Pharmacol, 13*, 990505, https://doi.org/10.3389/fphar.2022.990505.
48. Liu, Y., Wang, J., Zhang, M., Li, H., & Lin, Z. (2020). Polymer-Ligated Nanocrystals Enabled by Nonlinear Block Copolymer Nanoreactors: Synthesis, Properties, and Applications. *ACS Nano, 14*(10), 12491–12521, https://doi.org/10.1021/acsnano.0c06936.
49. Kamaly, N., Yameen, B., Wu, J., & Farokhzad, O. C. (2016). Degradable Controlled-Release Polymers and Polymeric Nanoparticles: Mechanisms of Controlling Drug Release. *Chemical Reviews, 116*(4), 2602–2663, https://doi.org/10.1021/acs.chemrev.5b00346.
50. Fernandes, A. I., & Jozala, A. F. (2022). Polymers Enhancing Bioavailability in Drug Delivery. *Pharmaceutics, 14*(10), https://doi.org/10.3390/pharmaceutics14102199.
51. Ullah, A., Marina, K., Yibang, Z., Muhammad, S., Mohsan, U., Azar, A., et al. (2025). Advancing Therapeutic Strategies with Polymeric Drug Conjugates for Nucleic Acid Delivery and Treatment. *International Journal of Nanomedicine, 20*(null), 25–52, https://doi.org/10.2147/IJN.S429279.
52. Spada, A., & Gerber-Lemaire, S. (2025). Surface Functionalization of Nanocarriers with Anti-EGFR Ligands for Cancer Active Targeting. *Nanomaterials (Basel), 15*(3), https://doi.org/10.3390/nano15030158.
53. Attia, M. F., Anton, N., Wallyn, J., Omran, Z., & Vandamme, T. F. (2019). An overview of active and passive targeting strategies to improve the nanocarriers efficiency to tumour sites. *Journal of Pharmacy and Pharmacology, 71*(8), 1185–1198, https://doi.org/10.1111/jphp.13098.
54. Martin, C., Aibani, N., Callan, J. F., & Callan, B. (2016). Recent advances in amphiphilic polymers for simultaneous delivery of hydrophobic and hydrophilic drugs. *Ther Deliv, 7*(1), 15–31, https://doi.org/10.4155/tde.15.84.
55. Austria, E., Bilek, M., Varamini, P., & Akhavan, B. (2025). Breaking biological barriers: Engineering polymeric nanoparticles for cancer therapy. *Nano Today, 60*, 102552, https://doi.org/10.1016/j.nantod.2024.102552.

56. Li, W., Tang, J., Lee, D., Tice, T. R., Schwendeman, S. P., & Prausnitz, M. R. (2022). Clinical translation of long-acting drug delivery formulations. *Nature Reviews Materials, 7*(5), 406–420, https://doi.org/10.1038/s41578-021-00405-w.
57. Kim, Y. M., Lee, Y. S., Kim, T., Yang, K., Nam, K., Choe, D., et al. (2020). Cationic cellulose nanocrystals complexed with polymeric siRNA for efficient anticancer drug delivery. *Carbohydrate Polymers, 247*, 116684, https://doi.org/10.1016/j.carbpol.2020.116684.
58. Yenurkar, D., Nayak, M., & Mukherjee, S. (2023). Recent advances of nanocrystals in cancer theranostics. *Nanoscale Adv, 5*(16), 4018–4040, https://doi.org/10.1039/d3na00397c.
59. Kumar, M., Jha, A., Goswami, P., Srivastava, R., Manjit, M., Bharti, K., et al. (2025). Fabrication of lipid-modified drug nanocrystals loaded injectable hydrogel for breast cancer therapy. *Discover Nano, 20*(1), 30, https://doi.org/10.1186/s11671-025-04195-w.
60. Gandhi, S., & Shastri, D. H. (2024). WITHDRAWN: Lipid-based Nanoparticulate Drug Delivery. *Pharm Nanotechnol*, https://doi.org/10.2174/0122117385275514231127062730.
61. Yap, S. L., Dyett, B., Hobro, A. J., Nguyen, H., Smith, N. I., Drummond, C. J., et al. (2025). The Internal Nanostructure of Lipid Nanoparticles Influences Their Diverse Cellular Uptake Pathways. *Small, n/a*(n/a), 2500903, https://doi.org/10.1002/smll.202500903.
62. Nsairat, H., Khater, D., Sayed, U., Odeh, F., Al Bawab, A., & Alshaer, W. (2022). Liposomes: structure, composition, types, and clinical applications. *Heliyon, 8*(5), e09394, https://doi.org/10.1016/j.heliyon.2022.e09394.
63. Akanda, M., Mithu, M. D. S. H., & Douroumis, D. (2023). Solid lipid nanoparticles: An effective lipid-based technology for cancer treatment. *Journal of Drug Delivery Science and Technology, 86*, 104709, https://doi.org/10.1016/j.jddst.2023.104709.
64. M, N. K., S, S., P, S. R., & Narayanasamy, D. (2024). The Science of Solid Lipid Nanoparticles: From Fundamentals to Applications. *Cureus, 16*(9), e68807, https://doi.org/10.7759/cureus.68807.
65. Sri Rekha, M., Sangeetha, S., & Seetha Devi, A. (2023). Solid Lipid Nanoparticles: A Potential Option for Enhancing Oral Bioavailability of Highly Soluble and Poorly Permeable (BCS Class III) Drugs. *Curr Drug Deliv, 20*(3), 223–236, https://doi.org/10.2174/1567201819666220418100410.
66. Peng, X., Fang, J., Lou, C., Yang, L., Shan, S., Wang, Z., et al. (2024). Engineered nanoparticles for precise targeted drug delivery and enhanced therapeutic efficacy in cancer immunotherapy. *Acta Pharmaceutica Sinica B, 14*(8), 3432–3456, https://doi.org/10.1016/j.apsb.2024.05.010.
67. Mehta, M., Bui, T. A., Yang, X., Aksoy, Y., Goldys, E. M., & Deng, W. (2023). Lipid-Based Nanoparticles for Drug/Gene Delivery: An Overview of the Production Techniques and Difficulties Encountered in Their Industrial Development. *ACS Materials Au, 3*(6), 600–619, https://doi.org/10.1021/acsmaterialsau.3c00032.
68. Dhayalan, M., Wang, W., Riyaz, S. U. M., Dinesh, R. A., Shanmugam, J., Irudayaraj, S. S., et al. (2024). Advances in functional lipid nanoparticles: from drug delivery platforms to clinical applications. *3 Biotech, 14*(2), 57, https://doi.org/10.1007/s13205-023-03901-8.
69. Shah, R. M., Jadhav, S. R., Bryant, G., Kaur, I. P., & Harding, I. H. (2025). On the formation and stability mechanisms of diverse lipid-based nanostructures for drug delivery. *Advances in Colloid and Interface Science, 338*, 103402, https://doi.org/10.1016/j.cis.2025.103402.
70. Chauhan, I., Yasir, M., Verma, M., & Singh, A. P. (2020). Nanostructured Lipid Carriers: A Groundbreaking Approach for Transdermal Drug Delivery. *Adv Pharm Bull, 10*(2), 150–165, https://doi.org/10.34172/apb.2020.021.
71. Panwar, P., Kumar, S., Chand, P., Chauhan, A. S., & Jakhmola, V. (2025). Nanostructured lipid carriers (NLCs): A comprehensive review of drug delivery advancements. *Journal of Applied Pharmaceutical Research, 13*(2), 20–38, https://doi.org/10.69857/joapr.v13i2.676.

72. Öztürk, K., Kaplan, M., & Çalış, S. (2024). Effects of nanoparticle size, shape, and zeta potential on drug delivery. *International Journal of Pharmaceutics, 666*, 124799, https://doi.org/10.1016/j.ijpharm.2024.124799.
73. Parvin, N., Joo, S. W., & Mandal, T. K. (2025). Biodegradable and Stimuli-Responsive Nanomaterials for Targeted Drug Delivery in Autoimmune Diseases. *Journal of Functional Biomaterials, 16*(1), 24.
74. Singh, P., Pandit, S., Balusamy, S. R., Madhusudanan, M., Singh, H., Amsath Haseef, H. M., et al. (2025). Advanced Nanomaterials for Cancer Therapy: Gold, Silver, and Iron Oxide Nanoparticles in Oncological Applications. *Advanced Healthcare Materials, 14*(4), 2403059, https://doi.org/10.1002/adhm.202403059.
75. Lankoff, A. M., Czerwińska, M., & Kruszewski, M. (2024). Advances in Nanotheranostic Systems for Concurrent Cancer Imaging and Therapy: An Overview of the Last 5 Years. *Molecules, 29*(24), 5985.
76. Wang, B., Hu, S., Teng, Y., Chen, J., Wang, H., Xu, Y., et al. (2024). Current advance of nanotechnology in diagnosis and treatment for malignant tumors. *Signal Transduction and Targeted Therapy, 9*(1), 200, https://doi.org/10.1038/s41392-024-01889-y.
77. Patel, A., Patel, K., Patel, V., Rajput, M. S., Patel, R., & Rajput, A. (2024). Nanocrystals: an emerging paradigm for cancer therapeutics. *Future Journal of Pharmaceutical Sciences, 10*(1), 4, https://doi.org/10.1186/s43094-024-00579-4.
78. Juan, A., Segrelles, C., del Campo-Balguerías, A., Bravo, I., Silva, I., Peral, J., et al. (2023). Anti-EGFR conjugated nanoparticles to deliver Alpelisib as targeted therapy for head and neck cancer. *Cancer Nanotechnology, 14*(1), 29, https://doi.org/10.1186/s12645-023-00180-z.
79. Aboushoushah, S. F. O. (2025). Iron oxide nanoparticles enhancing magnetic resonance imaging: A review of the latest advancements. *Journal of Science: Advanced Materials and Devices, 10*(2), 100875, https://doi.org/10.1016/j.jsamd.2025.100875.
80. Savari, M.-N., & Jabali, A. (2023). Properties of Iron Oxide Nanoparticles (IONPs). In M.-N. Savari, & A. Jabali (Eds.), *Theranostic Iron-Oxide Based Nanoplatforms in Oncology: Synthesis, Metabolism, and Toxicity for Simultaneous Imaging and Therapy* (pp. 49–65). Singapore: Springer Nature Singapore.
81. Sun, J.-P., Ren, Y.-T., Wei, K., He, M.-J., Gao, B.-H., & Qi, H. (2022). Photoacoustic response optimization of gold nanorods in the near-infrared region. *Results in Physics, 34*, 105209, https://doi.org/10.1016/j.rinp.2022.105209.
82. Abdellatif, A. A. H., Younis, M. A., Alsharidah, M., Al Rugaie, O., & Tawfeek, H. M. (2022). Biomedical Applications of Quantum Dots: Overview, Challenges, and Clinical Potential. *Int J Nanomedicine, 17*, 1951-1970, https://doi.org/10.2147/ijn.S357980.
83. Jiang, Z., Zhang, M., Li, P., Wang, Y., & Fu, Q. (2023). Nanomaterial-based CT contrast agents and their applications in image-guided therapy. *Theranostics, 13*(2), 483-509, https://doi.org/10.7150/thno.79625.
84. Kanal, E., Maki, J. H., Schramm, P., & Marti-Bonmati, L. (2025). Evolving Characteristics of Gadolinium-Based Contrast Agents for MR Imaging: A Systematic Review of the Importance of Relaxivity. *Journal of Magnetic Resonance Imaging, 61*(1), 52–69, https://doi.org/10.1002/jmri.29367.
85. Chow, J. C. L. (2025). Nanomaterial-Based Molecular Imaging in Cancer: Advances in Simulation and AI Integration. *Biomolecules, 15*(3), 444.
86. Bao, G., Mitragotri, S., & Tong, S. (2013). Multifunctional nanoparticles for drug delivery and molecular imaging. *Annu Rev Biomed Eng, 15*, 253–282, https://doi.org/10.1146/annurev-bioeng-071812-152409.

## References

87. Avasthi, A., Caro, C., Pozo-Torres, E., Leal, M. P., & García-Martín, M. L. (2020). Magnetic Nanoparticles as MRI Contrast Agents. *Top Curr Chem (Cham), 378*(3), 40, https://doi.org/10.1007/s41061-020-00302-w.
88. Puccetti, M., Pariano, M., Schoubben, A., Giovagnoli, S., & Ricci, M. (2024). Biologics, theranostics, and personalized medicine in drug delivery systems. *Pharmacological Research, 201*, 107086, https://doi.org/10.1016/j.phrs.2024.107086.
89. Singh, V. (2024). Theranostics: Integrated Diagnostics and Therapy Using Nanomedicine. In V. Gautam, R. Kumar, K. Das Manandhar, & S. C. Kamble (Eds.), *Nanomedicine: Innovations, Applications, and Breakthroughs in the Quest for Health and Medicine's Future* (pp. 505–530). Cham: Springer Nature Switzerland.
90. Guo, Z., Yu, G., Zhang, Z., Han, Y., Guan, G., Yang, W., et al. (2023). Intrinsic Optical Properties and Emerging Applications of Gold Nanostructures. *Advanced Materials, 35*(23), 2206700, https://doi.org/10.1002/adma.202206700.
91. Yang, W., Liang, H., Ma, S., Wang, D., & Huang, J. (2019). Gold nanoparticle based photothermal therapy: Development and application for effective cancer treatment. *Sustainable Materials and Technologies, 22*, e00109, https://doi.org/10.1016/j.susmat.2019.e00109.
92. Vines, J. B., Yoon, J. H., Ryu, N. E., Lim, D. J., & Park, H. (2019). Gold Nanoparticles for Photothermal Cancer Therapy. *Front Chem, 7*, 167, https://doi.org/10.3389/fchem.2019.00167.
93. Agostinis, P., Berg, K., Cengel, K. A., Foster, T. H., Girotti, A. W., Gollnick, S. O., et al. (2011). Photodynamic therapy of cancer: An update. *CA: A Cancer Journal for Clinicians, 61*(4), 250–281, https://doi.org/10.3322/caac.20114.
94. Ancély Ferreira dos, S., Daria Raquel Queiroz de, A., Leticia Ferreira, T., Maurício, S. B., & Leticia, L. (2019). Photodynamic therapy in cancer treatment - an update review. *Journal of Cancer Metastasis and Treatment, 5*, 25, https://doi.org/10.20517/2394-4722.2018.83.
95. Overchuk, M., Weersink, R. A., Wilson, B. C., & Zheng, G. (2023). Photodynamic and Photothermal Therapies: Synergy Opportunities for Nanomedicine. *ACS Nano, 17*(9), 7979–8003, https://doi.org/10.1021/acsnano.3c00891.
96. Merlin, J. P. J., Crous, A., & Abrahamse, H. (2024). Combining Photodynamic Therapy and Targeted Drug Delivery Systems: Enhancing Mitochondrial Toxicity for Improved Cancer Outcomes. *Int J Mol Sci, 25*(19), https://doi.org/10.3390/ijms251910796.
97. Vangijzegem, T., Lecomte, V., Ternad, I., Van Leuven, L., Muller, R. N., Stanicki, D., et al. (2023). Superparamagnetic Iron Oxide Nanoparticles (SPION): From Fundamentals to State-of-the-Art Innovative Applications for Cancer Therapy. *Pharmaceutics, 15*(1), https://doi.org/10.3390/pharmaceutics15010236.
98. Farzin, A., Etesami, S. A., Quint, J., Memic, A., & Tamayol, A. (2020). Magnetic Nanoparticles in Cancer Therapy and Diagnosis. *Adv Healthc Mater, 9*(9), e1901058, https://doi.org/10.1002/adhm.201901058.
99. Mukhatov, A., Le, T.-A., Pham, T. T., & Do, T. D. (2023). A comprehensive review on magnetic imaging techniques for biomedical applications. *Nano Select, 4*(3), 213–230, https://doi.org/10.1002/nano.202200219.
100. Chenxi, Z., Hemmat, A., Thi, N. H., & Afrand, M. (2025). Nanoparticle-enhanced drug delivery systems: An up-to-date review. *Journal of Molecular Liquids, 424*, 126999, https://doi.org/10.1016/j.molliq.2025.126999.
101. Delille, F., Pu, Y., Lequeux, N., & Pons, T. (2022). Designing the Surface Chemistry of Inorganic Nanocrystals for Cancer Imaging and Therapy. *Cancers (Basel), 14*(10), https://doi.org/10.3390/cancers14102456.
102. Shen, Y., Sun, Y., Yan, R., Chen, E., Wang, H., Ye, D., et al. (2017). Rational engineering of semiconductor QDs enabling remarkable 1O2 production for tumor-targeted photodynamic therapy. *Biomaterials, 148*, 31–40, https://doi.org/10.1016/j.biomaterials.2017.09.026.

103. Chen, Y., Yang, J., Fu, S., & Wu, J. (2020). Gold Nanoparticles as Radiosensitizers in Cancer Radiotherapy. *Int J Nanomedicine, 15*, 9407–9430, https://doi.org/10.2147/ijn.S272902.
104. Shi, S., Zhong, H., Zhang, Y., & Mei, Q. (2024). Targeted delivery of nano-radiosensitizers for tumor radiotherapy. *Coordination Chemistry Reviews, 518*, 216101, https://doi.org/10.1016/j.ccr.2024.216101.
105. Ayoubi, M., Naserzadeh, P., Hashemi, M. T., Reza Rostami, M., Tamjid, E., Tavakoli, M. M., et al. (2017). Biochemical mechanisms of dose-dependent cytotoxicity and ROS-mediated apoptosis induced by lead sulfide/graphene oxide quantum dots for potential bioimaging applications. *Scientific Reports, 7*(1), 12896, https://doi.org/10.1038/s41598-017-13396-y.
106. Gurunathan, S., Kang, M. H., Qasim, M., & Kim, J. H. (2018). Nanoparticle-Mediated Combination Therapy: Two-in-One Approach for Cancer. *Int J Mol Sci, 19*(10), https://doi.org/10.3390/ijms19103264.
107. Wang, H., & Huang, Y. (2020). Combination therapy based on nano codelivery for overcoming cancer drug resistance. *Medicine in Drug Discovery, 6*, 100024, https://doi.org/10.1016/j.medidd.2020.100024.

# Immunomodulation, Immunotherapy, Biotherapeutics Through Nanocrystals

Cancer continues to pose a significant universal health threat, with elevated illness and death rates despite innovations in early recognition and therapeutic interventions [1, 2]. In the current era, the field of tumor immunology has reshaped malignancy treatment paradigms by leveraging the host defense mechanisms to recognize and destroy tumor cells [3–5]. Approaches like, tumor immune evasion mediator blockade, cytokine therapy, oncologic vaccines, and adoptive engineered cell therapies have demonstrated profound and durable clinical responses in various malignancies [3, 6, 7]. However, these immunotherapeutic approaches are often hindered by several limitations, including poor bioavailability, off-target toxicity, short systemic half-lives, and immune suppression within the tumor microenvironment (TME) [8–10].

Immunomodulation, the deliberate regulation of immune responses, provides a versatile framework for overcoming these barriers [11, 12]. It encompasses both immune stimulation to enhance antitumor activity and immunosuppression to mitigate adverse immune reactions [13–15]. The effectiveness of immunomodulation in cancer depends critically on the precise delivery of immunostimulatory or immunosuppressive agents to the appropriate cellular targets within the TME or lymphoid organs [16–20].

The emergence of nanotechnology, and specifically nanocrystal-based delivery systems, has provided powerful tools to address the delivery challenges associated with immunotherapeutics [21–23]. Nanocrystals are pure drug particles engineered at the nanometer scale, typically stabilized with biocompatible surfactants or polymers [23–25]. Unlike traditional nanocarriers, nanocrystals are composed almost entirely of the active pharmaceutical ingredient, offering unmatched active ingredient loading and augmented solubility for weakly water-soluble compounds [24, 25].

Nanocrystals also offer the potential for both diagnostic imaging and therapeutic delivery within a single platform [26]. Their surfaces can be engineered to display targeting ligands or conjugated with imaging moieties, including fluorescent probes, MRI contrast materials, or radionuclides [26–28]. This enables instantaneous tracking of whole-body distribution, tumor localization, and immune cell engagement while simultaneously exerting therapeutic effects [28, 29]. For example, nanocrystals loaded with immunostimulatory agents can be directed toward tumor-resident dendritic cells, priming systemic immune responses, while also being visualized via noninvasive imaging modalities [30, 31].

Moreover, nanocrystals facilitate combination immunotherapy approaches by enabling co-delivery of chemotherapeutics, checkpoint inhibitors, or cancer vaccines in a spatially and temporally controlled manner [32–35]. These multifunctional systems are particularly valuable in creating an in situ vaccine effect, whereby tumor cell death induced by cytotoxic agents is coupled with immune activation, converting the tumor into its own source of antigens [36].

This chapter focuses on the engineering, functional tailoring, and deployment of nanocrystal-based platforms for cancer immunomodulation, immunotherapy, and biotherapeutics, with a focus on their role in theranostic strategies. We will discuss the advantages of nanocrystals in delivering immune agents, highlight their integration with imaging technologies, and examine preclinical and translational advances that position them as promising candidates for next-generation personalized oncology.

## 4.1 Design Principles of Nanocrystal Formulations

The fundamental material attributes of nanocrystals, like size profile, surface exposure ratio, crystallinity, polymorphism, and surface charge, control their therapeutic efficacy [37, 38]. All of which directly influence solubility, dissolution rate, and in vivo pharmacokinetics [39]. Acquiring knowledge of these factors is central to optimizing nanocrystal stability, drug release kinetics, and biological interactions [40–42]. Additionally, the influence of stabilizers such as surfactants and polymers in preventing aggregation and enhancing circulation time [43, 44]. The quality-by-design principles in measurement approaches, including those that enhance surface modification of nanocrystals, also improve biological performance and targeting efficiency [45]. Techniques such as PEGylation improve systemic circulation by reducing recognition by immune factors and subsezzquent clearance by the reticuloendothelial system [46, 47]. Notably, active targeting strategies involve the conjugation of targeting agents, including small peptides, antibodies, and small molecules such as folate, that bind to receptors aberrantly expressed in cancer cells surface or tumor-associated immunocytes, enhancing the selective distribution efficiency [48–50]. Co-surface loading with immunomodulators or adjuvants can further potentiate immune activation [51, 52]. Additionally, the integration of diagnostic agents, such as near-infrared dyes for optical imaging, gadolinium-based agents for magnetic resonance imaging, and radioactive probes for positron and single-photon emission tomography, is also important [53, 54]. Methods for covalent and non-covalent attachment of imaging moieties are examined to enable the development of multifunctional theranostic nanocrystals [55].

## 4.2 Nanocrystal-Mediated Delivery of Immunomodulators and Biotherapeutics

The integration of nanocrystal platforms into immunotherapy is gaining significant momentum, primarily due to their unique ability to enhance the distribution, stability, and biological availability of immunologically active agents [23, 56]. These platforms have demonstrated significant potential in transporting a widespread range of immune modulators, including Toll-like receptor (TLR) agonists such as imiquimod and resiquimod, which stimulate innate immune responses [57]. They are also being employed to deliver stimulators of interferon genes agonists that activate cytoplasmic DNA recognition pathways, triggering robust production of type I interferons [58, 59]. Additionally, nanocrystals are utilized for the targeted transport of small-molecule immune checkpoint inhibitors, aiming to recover T-cell functionality within the tumor milieu [60, 61]. Immune-modulating cytokines benefit from nanocrystal encapsulation by achieving sustained release and reduced systemic toxicity [62]. Moreover, nanocrystal platforms facilitate the efficient presentation of tumor-associated antigens, enhancing antigen-precise immune responses and supporting the development of personalized cancer vaccines [63, 64]. This emerging approach is poised to transform the realm of cancer immunotherapy via improvement of the pharmacokinetics, targeting precision, and therapeutic efficacy of diverse immunomodulatory agents [3, 13]. Nanocrystals enhance the solubility and cellular uptake of these agents, facilitating lymphatic transport to key immune organs, including lymph nodes and the spleen [16, 65–67]. The nanocrystals can co-deliver combinations of immunomodulators with chemotherapeutics or checkpoint inhibitors to achieve synergistic antitumor effects and modulate the immunosuppressive tumor microenvironment [68, 69]. The tumor microenvironment (TME) is characterized by immune evasion, chronic inflammation, and immunosuppressive signaling [70]. Nanocrystal-based immunomodulators address these hallmarks by enhancing the delivery of TLR or STING agonists to APCs, sustaining the release of cytokine mimetics, co-delivering antigens and adjuvants for in situ vaccination, and targeting immunoregulatory cells like MDSCs and Tregs [71, 72]. For example, Nanocrystals of a TLR7/8 agonist (e.g., resiquimod) conjugated with tumor-targeting ligands result in the selective uptake of these ligands by intratumoral dendritic cells, thereby enhancing antigen presentation and subsequent T-cell infiltration.

## 4.3 Theranostic Integration: Imaging-Guided Immune Activation

Nanocrystal systems offer a unique dual functionality by combining therapeutic efficacy with diagnostic imaging capabilities, making them powerful tools for cancer theranostics [26, 73]. Advanced strategies have been developed to integrate various imaging agents directly into nanocrystal constructs [27, 28, 74]. These include the incorporation of fluorescent dyes for optical imaging contrast-enhancing agents for MRI, and computed tomography (CT)-active metals like gold for enhanced radiographic contrast [75, 76]. Additionally, positron emission tomography (PET) tracers can be embedded to enable highly sensitive, real-time tracking of nanocrystal biodistribution and tumor localization [77]. This multifunctional design enables simultaneous treatment and monitoring, facilitating precise, image-guided therapy and live analysis of therapeutic response [78]. The role of these multifunctional nanocrystals in real-time monitoring of immune activation, payload release kinetics, tumor accumulation, and therapeutic rejoinder is illustrated with preclinical cancer models [79]. Imaging-guided delivery not only improves precision but also enables dynamic evaluation of treatment efficacy, offering critical insights into patient-specific responses [80].

### 4.3.1 Diagnostic Component

Theranostic nanocrystals can be engineered to incorporate imaging agents such as: Iron oxide nanoparticles for MRI [81], fluorescent dyes (e.g., Cy5.5, ICG) for optical imaging [82, 83], radioisotopes (e.g., $^{64}$Cu, $^{125}$I) for PET/SPECT [84], gold nanoparticles for CT and photoacoustic imaging [28, 85, 86]. These enable Pre-therapy tumor localization, in vivo biodistribution mapping, Therapy response monitoring, and Real-time immune cell tracking [26, 87].

### 4.3.2 Therapeutic Component

Nanocrystals can deliver chemotherapeutics, such as paclitaxel and doxorubicin, as well as immune checkpoint modulators, including small-molecule PD-L1 inhibitors, cytokines, or nucleic acids for immune activation [88–91]. For example, Fig. 4.1 comprehensively demonstrates the strong therapeutic value of the PTX/DEC-NPs-αPD-L1 nanoplatform in addressing the major therapeutic hurdles in triple-negative breast cancer (TNBC), including chemoresistance, high metastatic potential, and poor prognosis [92].

## 4.3 Theranostic Integration: Imaging-Guided Immune Activation

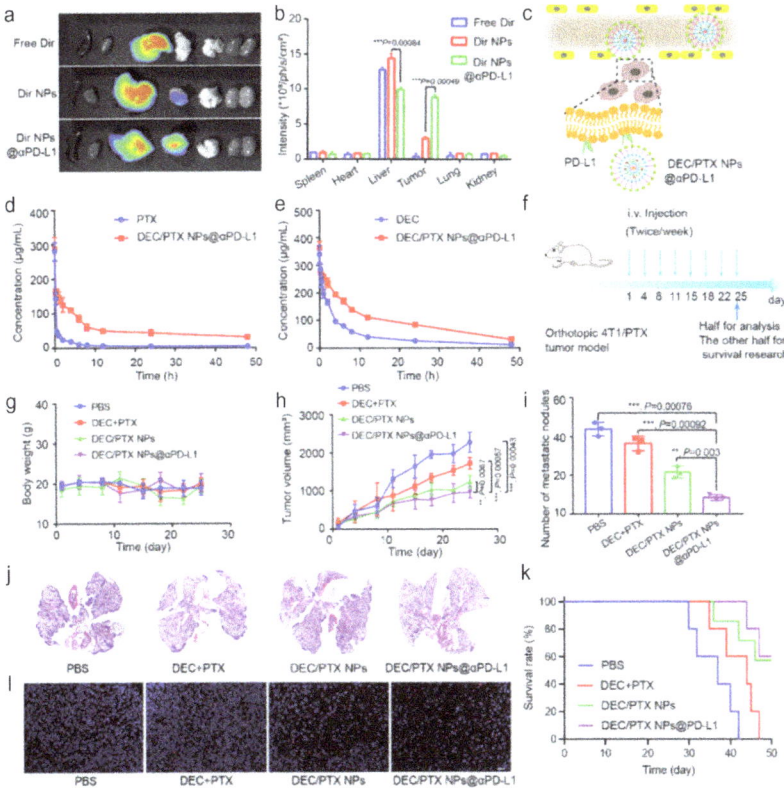

**Fig. 4.1** PTX/DEC-NPs-αPD-L1 actively target the tumor-specific region and markedly suppress both primary tumor growth and metastatic progression in a TNBC model. **a** In vivo fluorescence imaging showing distribution profile of free DiR dye, DiR-loaded nanoparticles (DiR NPs), and αPD-L1-conjugated DiR nanoparticles (DiR NPs-αPD-L1) in tumor-bearing mice. **b** Quantitative fluorescence analysis from major organs and tumor tissue confirms enhanced tumor accumulation with αPD-L1-targeted nanoparticles. **c** Schematic representation of the dual-targeting strategy: passive localization leveraging the EPR phenomenon, and active targeting through αPD-L1-mediated binding to PD-L1-expressing cancer cells. **d, e** Pharmacokinetic profiles of DEC (**d**) and PTX (**e**) in plasma following administration of PTX/DEC-NPs-αPD-L1 versus free drug formulations, analyzed by HPLC. F) Experimental timeline for intervention in an orthotopic 4T1/PTX breast tumor model in BALB/c mice, including dosing schedule and endpoint analyses. **g** Body mass monitoring of mice across treatment groups to assess systemic toxicity. **h** Tumor growth curves showing significant tumor suppression in mice dosed with PTX/DEC-NPs-αPD-L1 (n = 6). **i** Quantification of metastatic lung nodules indicates a substantial reduction in metastatic burden in the PTX/DEC-NPs-αPD-L1 group. **j** Representative H&E-stained lung sections from each treatment group confirm histological differences in metastatic spread. **k** Kaplan–Meier survival curves showing prolonged survival in mice treated with PTX/DEC-NPs-αPD-L1. **l** TUNEL staining of tumor sections reveals increased apoptosis in the PTX/DEC-NPs-αPD-L1 group. Scale bar: 100 μm. Data are expressed as mean ± SD. Statistical significance was dogged as follows: *P < 0.05, **P < 0.01, ***P < 0.001. Figure adapted from a recently published paper [92]

By co-delivering the DNA methyltransferase inhibitor decitabine (DEC) and the chemotherapeutic agent paclitaxel (PTX) within a nanoparticle modified with an anti-PD-L1 antibody, this system achieves a multifaceted therapeutic effect. The αPD-L1 modification enables precise targeting of PD-L1-expressing TNBC cells, enhancing tumor accumulation and facilitating immune checkpoint blockade. Once internalized, DEC epigenetically reprograms tumor cells by inhibiting DNMT1, shifting mesenchymal cells back to an epithelial state, reducing cancer stem cell populations, and restoring PTX sensitivity. Simultaneously, PTX induces direct cytotoxicity, disrupts the immunosuppressive tumor microenvironment, and promotes immunogenic cell death. Together, these mechanisms act synergistically to impede primary cancer growth, reduce metastatic spread, and advance overall endurance. This integrated strategy of tumor-specific delivery, immune activation, and dual-drug synergy presents a powerful and innovative approach for synchronizing chemoimmunotherapy in aggressive, treatment-resistant malignancies, such as TNBC [92].

## 4.4 Preclinical Applications of Theranostic Nanocrystals

Nanocrystals are being explored as tools to transform tumors into localized vaccine depots by creating immunologically active niches [93]. This approach involves: Co-delivering tumor-associated antigens (TAAs) or neoantigens with adjuvants, incorporating imaging tracers to monitor vaccine deposition and immune cell recruitment, and inducing local inflammation to enhance immune infiltration [94]. Nanocrystals co-loaded with tumor antigens, adjuvants, and microbubble contrast agents have demonstrated dual functionality, enabling both tumor imaging and synchronized immune activation in melanoma models [95]. Another example includes HER2-targeted nanocrystals that have been industrialized to co-deliver doxorubicin and checkpoint blockade agents, displaying added therapeutic efficacy in HER2-positive tumor models [96]. Similarly, STING-agonist-loaded nanocrystals have been shown to remodel the immunosuppressive microenvironment in pancreatic tumors, thereby promoting robust antitumor immune responses [97]. This study presents the development and evaluation of NMSR, a multifunctional nanotherapeutic platform co-delivering the STING pathway activator MSA-2 and STAT3 pathway inhibitor stattic, with iRGD-facilitated tumor targeting. The NMSR nanoparticles exhibit uniform spherical morphology and favorable size distribution [97]. In vitro assays demonstrate that NMSR exhibits enhanced cytotoxicity in cancer cells compared to untargeted or single-agent formulations [97]. Confocal imaging of 3D tumor spheroids reveals deeper penetration of NMSR, attributed to iRGD functionalization. Live animal and tissue-based fluorescence imaging confirm improved tumor localization and retention of NMSR [97]. Finally, therapeutic studies in KPC tumor-bearing mice show that NMSR significantly reduces tumor growth and improves survival, highlighting its

## 4.4 Preclinical Applications of Theranostic Nanocrystals

potential as an active immunotherapeutic nanoplatform for pancreatic tumor treatment [97].

In the context of glioma, brain-penetrant nanocrystals engineered to traverse the blood–brain barrier have enabled the effective delivery of immune modulators and checkpoint inhibitors, thereby enhancing immunotherapy outcomes [98, 99].

Figure 4.2 illustrates a comprehensive overview of numerous functionalized nanocarriers designed to cross the blood–brain barrier (BBB) and target glioma cells, as discussed in Wu et al. [99]. It highlights multiple nanoparticle platforms, such as lipid nanoparticles, micelles, polymers, gold nanoparticles (AuNPs), carbon-based nanostructures, and extracellular vesicles, that can be modified with targeting ligands and loaded with therapeutic agents. These nanocarriers are engineered to augment drug accumulation in glioma tissue while diminishing off-target effects [103]. The bottom section of the figure shows examples of surface-functionalized nanoparticles using ligands such as iRGD, c(RGDfK), Pep-22, VAP, and AP-2, which are tailored to specific receptors overexpressed at the BBB and within glioma cells. These constructs deliver a range of therapeutic drugs, as well as contrast agents or a combination of them, via strategies such as membrane coating, dual-ligand targeting, and superparamagnetic guidance. Overall, the figure underscores the adaptability and precision of nanoparticle-based delivery systems in overcoming the BBB and achieving targeted glioma therapy [103].

Key therapeutic outcomes highlighted in recent studies include significant inhibition of tumor growth, augmented migration of immune effectors like $CD^{8+}$ T cells and dendritic cells into the tumor microenvironment, detailed profiling of cytokine responses to assess immune activation, and the use of imaging-based strategies to monitor therapeutic progress in real-time. These parameters collectively offer a comprehensive assessment of nanomedicine efficacy in cancer immunotherapy [100–104]. Further, HER2-targeted doxorubicin nanocrystals co-loaded with the near-infrared dye enabled dual functionality by facilitating real-time imaging and promoting immune-mediated cytotoxicity in HER2-positive breast cancer models [105]. Additionally, PEGylated paclitaxel nanocarriers have demonstrated the ability to remodel the tumor stroma and reverse immune suppression, thereby enhancing the therapeutic effectiveness of the immune checkpoint barricade [106]. In preclinical studies, paclitaxel formulated into PEGylated nanomicelles retained its capacity to induce immunogenic cell death, leading to increased infiltration of cytotoxic T cells ($CD^{8+}$) and dendritic cells, which are localized within the tumor niche. When joint with anti–PD1 therapy, this method significantly enhanced antitumor responses by promoting a more immunostimulatory tumor microenvironment and overcoming resistance to checkpoint inhibition. These conclusions underscore the likelihood of nanocarrier-based combination strategies in potentiating cancer immunotherapy [106].

In summary, nanocrystal-based theranostics offer a transformative approach to cancer diagnosis and immunotherapy by integrating efficient drug delivery, precise immune modulation, and real-time imaging capabilities. These multifunctional platforms have

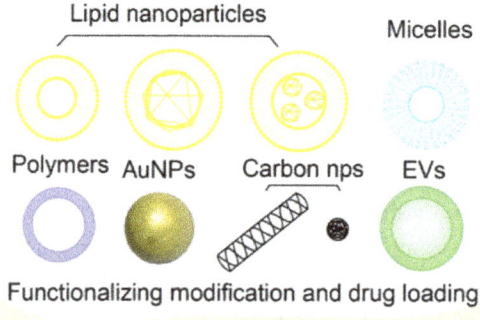
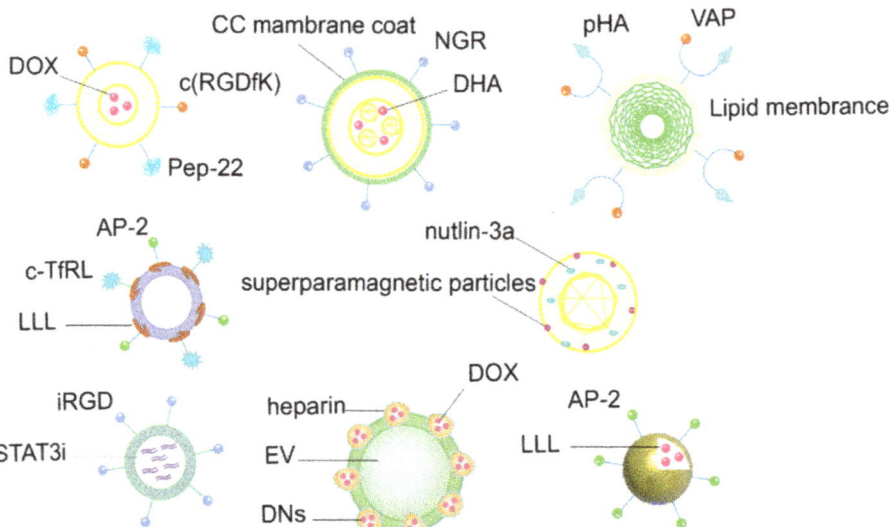

**Fig. 4.2** Nanoparticles with functionalizing modification and drug loading. The figure illustrates various nanocarriers like lipid-based NPs, micelles, polymers, AuNPs, carbon structures, and biomaterial-derived NPs engineered with targeting ligands and loaded with drugs to enable dual-targeting of the blood–brain barrier (BBB) and glioma cells [103]

the potential to significantly advance precision oncology by enabling targeted treatment and continuous monitoring of therapeutic outcomes. With ongoing interdisciplinary innovations aimed at addressing current challenges, the clinical translation of nanocrystal-based theranostic systems holds great promise for enhancing cancer detection, improving treatment response, and achieving sustained therapeutic benefits.

## References

1. Cai, Y., Dai, F., Ye, Y., & Qian, J. (2025). The global burden of breast cancer among women of reproductive age: a comprehensive analysis. *Scientific Reports, 15*(1), 9347.
2. Ahmad, I., Jasim, S. A., Sharma, M., S, R. J., Hjazi, A., Mohammed, J. S., et al. (2024). New paradigms to break barriers in early cancer detection for improved prognosis and treatment outcomes. *The Journal of Gene Medicine, 26*(8), e3730.
3. Raghani, N. R., Chorawala, M. R., Mahadik, M., Patel, R. B., Prajapati, B. G., & Parekh, P. S. (2024). Revolutionizing cancer treatment: Comprehensive insights into immunotherapeutic strategies. *Medical Oncology, 41*(2), 51.
4. Rezaei, N. (2023). *Cancer treatment: an interdisciplinary approach*: Springer.
5. Jain, K. K., & Jain, K. K. (2021). Personalized immuno-oncology. *Textbook of Personalized Medicine*, 479–508.
6. Kubli, S. P., Berger, T., Araujo, D. V., Siu, L. L., & Mak, T. W. (2021). Beyond immune checkpoint blockade: emerging immunological strategies. *Nature reviews Drug discovery, 20*(12), 899–919.
7. Liu, B., Zhou, H., Tan, L., Siu, K. T. H., & Guan, X.-Y. (2024). Exploring treatment options in cancer: tumor treatment strategies. *Signal transduction and targeted therapy, 9*(1), 175.
8. Manzari, M. T., Shamay, Y., Kiguchi, H., Rosen, N., Scaltriti, M., & Heller, D. A. (2021). Targeted drug delivery strategies for precision medicines. *Nature Reviews Materials, 6*(4), 351–370.
9. Nel, A. E., Mei, K.-C., Liao, Y.-P., & Liu, X. (2022). Multifunctional lipid bilayer nanocarriers for cancer immunotherapy in heterogeneous tumor microenvironments, combining immunogenic cell death stimuli with immune modulatory drugs. *ACS nano, 16*(4), 5184–5232.
10. Yu, L., Liu, S., Jia, S., & Xu, F. (2023). Emerging frontiers in drug delivery with special focus on novel techniques for targeted therapies. *Biomedicine & Pharmacotherapy, 165*, 115049.
11. Strzelec, M., Detka, J., Mieszczak, P., Sobocińska, M. K., & Majka, M. (2023). Immunomodulation—a general review of the current state-of-the-art and new therapeutic strategies for targeting the immune system. *Frontiers in Immunology, 14*, 1127704.
12. Singh, M. R., Yadav, K., Chaurasiya, N. D., & Singh, D. (2022). Immune system and mechanism of immunomodulation. In *Plants and Phytomolecules for Immunomodulation: Recent Trends and Advances* (pp. 1–31): Springer.
13. Kraehenbuehl, L., Weng, C.-H., Eghbali, S., Wolchok, J. D., & Merghoub, T. (2022). Enhancing immunotherapy in cancer by targeting emerging immunomodulatory pathways. *Nature reviews Clinical oncology, 19*(1), 37–50.
14. Czajka-Francuz, P., Prendes, M. J., Mankan, A., Quintana, A., Pabla, S., Ramkissoon, S., et al. (2023). Mechanisms of immune modulation in the tumor microenvironment and implications for targeted therapy. *Frontiers in Oncology, 13*, 1200646.
15. Bernitsa, S., Dayan, R., Stephanou, A., Tzvetanova, I. D., & Patrikios, I. S. (2023). Natural biomolecules and derivatives as anticancer immunomodulatory agents. *Frontiers in Immunology, 13*, 1070367.
16. Hsu, J. C., Liu, P., Song, Y., Song, W., Saladin, R. J., Peng, Y., et al. (2024). Lymphoid organ-targeted nanomaterials for immunomodulation of cancer, inflammation, and beyond. *Chemical Society Reviews*.
17. Liu, J., & Huang, J. (2024). Immunemodulation and Cancer. In *Anesthesia for Oncological Surgery* (pp. 17–25): Springer.

18. Xie, L., & Meng, Z. (2023). Immunomodulatory effect of locoregional therapy in the tumor microenvironment. *Molecular Therapy, 31*(4), 951–969.
19. Khatua, R., Bhar, B., Dey, S., Jaiswal, C., & Mandal, B. B. (2024). Advances in engineered nanosystems: immunomodulatory interactions for therapeutic applications. *Nanoscale, 16*(27), 12820–12856.
20. Sau, S., Dey, A., Pal, P., Das, B., Maity, K. K., Dash, S. K., et al. (2024). Immunomodulatory and immune-toxicological role of nanoparticles: Potential therapeutic applications. *International Immunopharmacology, 135*, 112251.
21. Gao, S., Yang, X., Xu, J., Qiu, N., & Zhai, G. (2021). Nanotechnology for boosting cancer immunotherapy and remodeling tumor microenvironment: the horizons in cancer treatment. *ACS nano, 15*(8), 12567–12603.
22. Wells, K., Liu, T., Zhu, L., & Yang, L. (2024). Immunomodulatory nanoparticles activate cytotoxic T cells for enhancement of the effect of cancer immunotherapy. *Nanoscale.*
23. Chary, P. S., Shaikh, S., Bhavana, V., Rajana, N., Vasave, R., & Mehra, N. K. (2024). Emerging role of nanocrystals in pharmaceutical applications: A review of regulatory aspects and drug development process. *Applied Materials Today, 40*, 102334.
24. Geng, F., Fan, X., Liu, Y., Lu, W., & Wei, G. (2024). Recent advances in nanocrystal-based technologies applied for ocular drug delivery. *Expert Opinion on Drug Delivery, 21*(2), 211–227.
25. Xue, L., Ding, J., Liu, Y., Ma, Y., Yang, C., Wang, W., et al. (2024). Strategies and methods of nanocrystal technology for targeting drug delivery. *Journal of Nanoparticle Research, 26*(6), 114.
26. Yenurkar, D., Nayak, M., & Mukherjee, S. (2023). Recent advances of nanocrystals in cancer theranostics. *Nanoscale Advances, 5*(16), 4018–4040.
27. Delille, F., Pu, Y., Lequeux, N., & Pons, T. (2022). Designing the surface chemistry of inorganic nanocrystals for cancer imaging and therapy. *Cancers, 14*(10), 2456.
28. Yang, Y., Jiang, Q., & Zhang, F. (2023). Nanocrystals for deep-tissue in vivo luminescence imaging in the near-infrared region. *Chemical Reviews, 124*(2), 554–628.
29. Kiani, M. N., Khaliq, H., Abubakar, M., Rafique, M., Jalilov, F., Ashraf, G. A., et al. (2025). Advancing the potential of nanoparticles for cancer detection and precision therapeutics. *Medical Oncology, 42*(7), 1–32.
30. Ma, M., Zhang, Y., Pu, K., & Tang, W. (2025). Nanomaterial-enabled metabolic reprogramming strategies for boosting antitumor immunity. *Chemical Society Reviews.*
31. Li, K., Zhang, Z., Mei, Y., Li, M., Yang, Q., Wu, Q., et al. (2022). Targeting the innate immune system with nanoparticles for cancer immunotherapy. *Journal of Materials Chemistry B, 10*(11), 1709–1733.
32. Kumbhar, P. R., Kumar, P., Lasure, A., Velayutham, R., & Mandal, D. (2023). An updated landscape on nanotechnology-based drug delivery, immunotherapy, vaccinations, imaging, and biomarker detections for cancers: Recent trends and future directions with clinical success. *Discover Nano, 18*(1), 156.
33. Dhas, N., Kudarha, R., Kulkarni, S., Soman, S., Navti, P. D., Kulkarni, J., et al. (2024). Nano-engineered Platform-Based Microenvironment-Triggered Immunotherapy in Cancer Treatment. *Frontiers in Bioscience-Landmark, 29*(10), 349.
34. Boone, C. E., Wang, L., Gautam, A., Newton, I. G., & Steinmetz, N. F. (2022). Combining nanomedicine and immune checkpoint therapy for cancer immunotherapy. *Wiley Interdisciplinary Reviews: Nanomedicine and Nanobiotechnology, 14*(1), e1739.
35. Nguyen, A., Kumar, S., & Kulkarni, A. A. (2022). Nanotheranostic strategies for cancer immunotherapy. *Small Methods, 6*(12), 2200718.

## References

36. Gong, N., Alameh, M.-G., El-Mayta, R., Xue, L., Weissman, D., & Mitchell, M. J. (2024). Enhancing in situ cancer vaccines using delivery technologies. *Nature reviews Drug discovery, 23*(8), 607–625, https://doi.org/10.1038/s41573-024-00974-9.
37. Pardhi, V. P., Verma, T., Flora, S., Chandasana, H., & Shukla, R. (2018). Nanocrystals: an overview of fabrication, characterization and therapeutic applications in drug delivery. *Current pharmaceutical design, 24*(43), 5129–5146.
38. Yanamadala, Y., Muthumula, C. M. R., Khare, S., & Gokulan, K. (2025). Strategies to Enhance Nanocrystal Formulations for Overcoming Physiological Barriers Across Diverse Routes of Administration. *International Journal of Nanomedicine, 20*(null), 367–402, https://doi.org/10.2147/IJN.S494224.
39. Manshi, Setya, S., & Talegaonkar, S. (2025). Advances and Developments in Formulation of Drug Nanocrystals. In K. Jain, & A. K. Yadav (Eds.), *Advances in Pharmaceutical Product Development* (pp. 321–354). Singapore: Springer Nature Singapore.
40. Gigliobianco, M. R., Casadidio, C., Censi, R., & Di Martino, P. (2018). Nanocrystals of poorly soluble drugs: drug bioavailability and physicochemical stability. *Pharmaceutics, 10*(3), 134.
41. Chogale, M. M., Ghodake, V. N., & Patravale, V. B. (2016). Performance parameters and characterizations of nanocrystals: A brief review. *Pharmaceutics, 8*(3), 26.
42. Chen, M.-L., John, M., Lee, S. L., & Tyner, K. M. (2017). Development considerations for nanocrystal drug products. *The AAPS journal, 19*, 642–651.
43. Tuomela, A., Hirvonen, J., & Peltonen, L. (2016). Stabilizing agents for drug nanocrystals: effect on bioavailability. *Pharmaceutics, 8*(2), 16.
44. Shete, G., Jain, H., Punj, D., Prajapat, H., Akotiya, P., & Bansal, A. K. (2016). Stabilizers used in nano-crystal based drug delivery systems. *International Journal of Pharmaceutical Excipients, 5*(4).
45. Zhao, J., Liu, Y., Wang, L., Zhou, Y., Du, J., & Wang, Y. (2018). Functional and modified nanocrystals technology for target drug delivery. *Journal of Nanoscience and Nanotechnology, 18*(8), 5207–5221.
46. Meyers, S. R., & Grinstaff, M. W. (2012). Biocompatible and bioactive surface modifications for prolonged in vivo efficacy. *Chemical Reviews, 112*(3), 1615–1632.
47. Kaminskas, L. M., & Boyd, B. J. (2011). Nanosized drug delivery vectors and the reticuloendothelial system. *Intracellular Delivery: Fundamentals and Applications*, 155–178.
48. Lu, Y., Sega, E., Leamon, C. P., & Low, P. S. (2004). Folate receptor-targeted immunotherapy of cancer: mechanism and therapeutic potential. *Advanced drug delivery reviews, 56*(8), 1161–1176.
49. Anarjan, F. S. (2019). Active targeting drug delivery nanocarriers: Ligands. *Nano-Structures & Nano-Objects, 19*, 100370.
50. Taghipour, Y. D., Zarebkohan, A., Salehi, R., Rahimi, F., Torchilin, V. P., Hamblin, M. R., et al. (2022). An update on dual targeting strategy for cancer treatment. *Journal of Controlled Release, 349*, 67–96.
51. Barchi Jr, J. J. (2022). Glycoconjugate nanoparticle-based systems in cancer immunotherapy: novel designs and recent updates. *Frontiers in Immunology, 13*, 852147.
52. Zhang, Y., Liu, L., He, H., Sun, Y., & Zhong, Z. (2024). Dual and multi-immune activation strategies for emerging cancer immunotherapy. *Materials Today, 80*, 406–428, https://doi.org/10.1016/j.mattod.2024.08.006.
53. Butt, A., & Bach, H. (2025). Advancements in nanotechnology for diagnostics: a literature review, part II: advanced techniques in nuclear and optical imaging. *Nanomedicine, 20*(2), 183–206.

54. He, J.-F., Yang, W.-W., Quan, W.-X., Yang, Y.-C., Zhang, Z., & Luo, Q.-Y. (2024). Application of rare earth elements in dual-modality molecular probes. *RSC advances, 14*(52), 38480–38490.
55. Hu, X. L., Kwon, N., Yan, K. C., Sedgwick, A. C., Chen, G. R., He, X. P., et al. (2020). Bio-Conjugated Advanced Materials for Targeted Disease Theranostics. *Advanced Functional Materials, 30*(13), 1907906.
56. Theivendren, P., Kunjiappan, S., Pavadai, P., Ravi, K., Murugavel, A., Dayalan, A., et al. (2024). Revolutionizing cancer immunotherapy: emerging nanotechnology-driven drug delivery systems for enhanced therapeutic efficacy. *ACS Measurement Science Au, 5*(1), 31–55.
57. Bhagchandani, S., Johnson, J. A., & Irvine, D. J. (2021). Evolution of Toll-like receptor 7/8 agonist therapeutics and their delivery approaches: From antiviral formulations to vaccine adjuvants. *Advanced drug delivery reviews, 175*, 113803.
58. Li, Y., Li, X., Yi, J., Cao, Y., Qin, Z., Zhong, Z., et al. (2023). Nanoparticle-mediated STING activation for cancer immunotherapy. *Advanced Healthcare Materials, 12*(19), 2300260.
59. Vasiyani, H. K. (2023). *Study of Expression of Cyclic-GMP-AMP Synthase (cGAS) and Stimulator of Interferon Genes (STING) in Breast Cancer and Its Potential for Anti-Cancer Therapy.* Maharaja Sayajirao University of Baroda (India).
60. Gao, S., Yang, D., Fang, Y., Lin, X., Jin, X., Wang, Q., et al. (2019). Engineering nanoparticles for targeted remodeling of the tumor microenvironment to improve cancer immunotherapy. *Theranostics, 9*(1), 126.
61. Tang, L., Mei, Y., Shen, Y., He, S., Xiao, Q., Yin, Y., et al. (2021). Nanoparticle-mediated targeted drug delivery to remodel tumor microenvironment for cancer therapy. *International Journal of Nanomedicine*, 5811–5829.
62. Holmberg, L., & Bensinger, W. (2006). Interleukin 2 (IL-2) and granulocyte-macrophage colony stimulating factor (sargramostin)(GM-CSF) following autologous peripheral blood stem cell transplant (ASCT) for breast cancer. *Biology of Blood and Marrow Transplantation, 12*(2), 98–99.
63. Guo, J., Liu, C., Qi, Z., Qiu, T., Zhang, J., & Yang, H. (2024). Engineering customized nanovaccines for enhanced cancer immunotherapy. *Bioactive Materials, 36*, 330–357.
64. Liang, J., & Zhao, X. (2021). Nanomaterial-based delivery vehicles for therapeutic cancer vaccine development. *Cancer Biology & Medicine, 18*(2), 352–371.
65. Tang, Y., Liu, B., Zhang, Y., Liu, Y., Huang, Y., & Fan, W. (2024). Interactions between nanoparticles and lymphatic systems: mechanisms and applications in drug delivery. *Advanced drug delivery reviews*, 115304.
66. Mhaske, A. S., & Shukla, R. (2023). Therapeutic Potential of Nanocrystals for Targeting Lymphoid Carcinoma. In *Handbook of Oncobiology: From Basic to Clinical Sciences* (pp. 1–21): Springer.
67. Chen, Y., De Koker, S., & De Geest, B. G. (2020). Engineering strategies for lymph node targeted immune activation. *Accounts of chemical research, 53*(10), 2055–2067.
68. Zhang, M.-R., Fang, L.-L., Guo, Y., Wang, Q., Li, Y.-J., Sun, H.-F., et al. (2024). Advancements in stimulus-responsive co-delivery nanocarriers for enhanced cancer immunotherapy. *International Journal of Nanomedicine*, 3387–3404.
69. Chen, Y., Sun, J., Huang, Y., Lu, B., & Li, S. (2018). Improved cancer immunochemotherapy via optimal co-delivery of chemotherapeutic and immunomodulatory agents. *Molecular pharmaceutics, 15*(11), 5162–5173.
70. Wang, D., & DuBois, R. N. (2015). Immunosuppression associated with chronic inflammation in the tumor microenvironment. *Carcinogenesis, 36*(10), 1085–1093.

71. Mohammad, I. S., Hu, H., Yin, L., & He, W. (2019). Drug nanocrystals: Fabrication methods and promising therapeutic applications. *International Journal of Pharmaceutics, 562*, 187–202, https://doi.org/10.1016/j.ijpharm.2019.02.045.
72. Zhang, J., Corpstein, C. D., & Li, T. (2021). Intracellular uptake of nanocrystals: Probing with aggregation-induced emission of fluorescence and kinetic modeling. *Acta Pharm Sin B, 11*(4), 1021–1029, https://doi.org/10.1016/j.apsb.2020.09.017.
73. Kelkar, S. S., & Reineke, T. M. (2011). Theranostics: combining imaging and therapy. *Bioconjugate chemistry, 22*(10), 1879–1903.
74. Cormode, D. P., Sanchez-Gaytan, B. L., Mieszawska, A. J., Fayad, Z. A., & Mulder, W. J. (2013). Inorganic nanocrystals as contrast agents in MRI: synthesis, coating and introduction of multifunctionality. *NMR in Biomedicine, 26*(7), 766–780.
75. Molkenova, A., Atabaev, T. S., Hong, S. W., Mao, C., Han, D.-W., & Kim, K. S. (2022). Designing inorganic nanoparticles into computed tomography and magnetic resonance (CT/MR) imaging-guidable photomedicines. *Materials Today Nano, 18*, 100187.
76. Neilio, J. M., & Ginat, D. T. (2024). Emerging Head and Neck Tumor Targeting Contrast Agents for the Purpose of CT, MRI, and Multimodal Diagnostic Imaging: A Molecular Review. *Diagnostics, 14*(15), 1666.
77. Polyak, A., & Ross, T. L. (2018). Nanoparticles for SPECT and PET imaging: towards personalized medicine and theranostics. *Current medicinal chemistry, 25*(34), 4328–4353.
78. Fernandez-Fernandez, A., Manchanda, R., & McGoron, A. J. (2011). Theranostic applications of nanomaterials in cancer: drug delivery, image-guided therapy, and multifunctional platforms. *Applied biochemistry and biotechnology, 165*, 1628–1651.
79. Patel, A., Patel, K., Patel, V., Rajput, M. S., Patel, R., & Rajput, A. (2024). Nanocrystals: an emerging paradigm for cancer therapeutics. *Future Journal of Pharmaceutical Sciences, 10*(1), 4.
80. Zhou, Q., Liu, Q., Wang, Y., Chen, J., Schmid, O., Rehberg, M., et al. (2024). Bridging smart nanosystems with clinically relevant models and advanced imaging for precision drug delivery. *Advanced science, 11*(14), 2308659.
81. Anani, T., Rahmati, S., Sultana, N., & David, A. E. (2021). MRI-traceable theranostic nanoparticles for targeted cancer treatment. *Theranostics, 11*(2), 579.
82. Russell, P., Velivolu, R., Maldonado Zimbrón, V., Hong, J., Kavianinia, I., Hickey, A., et al. (2022). Fluorescent tracers for in vivo imaging of lymphatic targets. *Frontiers in Pharmacology, 13*, 952581.
83. Rahiman, N. (2025). Updates and current states on liposomal vehicles for tumor targeting: precision therapy in the spotlight. *Cancer Nanotechnology, 16*(1), 12.
84. Shende, P., & Gandhi, S. (2021). Current strategies of radiopharmaceuticals in theranostic applications. *Journal of Drug Delivery Science and Technology, 64*, 102594.
85. Wu, J., Ko, S., Lee, E., Son, E., Kang, G., Hur, S., et al. (2025). Gold nanoparticles in imaging: advances, applications, and future perspectives. *Applied Spectroscopy Reviews*, 1–40.
86. Chen, J., Nguyen, V. P., Jaiswal, S., Kang, X., Lee, M., Paulus, Y. M., et al. (2021). Thin layer-protected gold nanoparticles for targeted multimodal imaging with photoacoustic and CT. *Pharmaceuticals, 14*(11), 1075.
87. Fernandes, D. A. (2023). Review on Metal-Based Theranostic Nanoparticles for Cancer Therapy and Imaging. *Technol Cancer Res Treat, 22*, 15330338231191493, https://doi.org/10.1177/15330338231191493.
88. Zhang, L., Zhu, C., Zhao, J., Scimeca, L., Dong, M., Liu, R., et al. (2024). Recent advances in nanomodulators for augmenting cancer immunotherapy in cold tumors: insights from drug delivery to drug-free strategies. *Advanced Functional Materials, 34*(18), 2311914.

89. Wang, X., Yin, X., Li, Y., Zhang, S., Hu, M., Wei, M., et al. (2024). Novel insight and perspectives of nanoparticle-mediated gene delivery and immune-modulating therapies for pancreatic cancer. *Journal of Nanobiotechnology, 22*(1), 771.
90. Li, J.-h., Huang, L.-j., Zhou, H.-l., Shan, Y.-m., Chen, F.-m., Lehto, V.-P., et al. (2022). Engineered nanomedicines block the PD-1/PD-L1 axis for potentiated cancer immunotherapy. *Acta Pharmacologica Sinica, 43*(11), 2749–2758.
91. Lang, X., Wang, X., Han, M., & Guo, Y. (2024). Nanoparticle-mediated synergistic chemoimmunotherapy for cancer treatment. *International Journal of Nanomedicine*, 4533–4568.
92. He, Y., Hu, Q., Wang, L., & Chen, C. (2024). Decitabine/paclitaxel co-delivery systems modified with anti-PD-L1 antibodies mediate chemoimmunotherapy for Triple negative breast cancer. *Materials & Design, 237*, 112562, https://doi.org/10.1016/j.matdes.2023.112562.
93. Aikins, M. E., Xu, C., & Moon, J. J. (2020). Engineered nanoparticles for cancer vaccination and immunotherapy. *Accounts of chemical research, 53*(10), 2094–2105.
94. Guo, C., Lin, L., Wang, Y., Jing, J., Gong, Q., & Luo, K. (2025). Nano drug delivery systems for advanced immune checkpoint blockade therapy. *Theranostics, 15*(11), 5440.
95. Elabed, S., Sheirf, A., & Ali, M. (2025). Nanostructures for cancer therapeutics and diagnostics: Recent advances and future outlook. *Radiation Physics and Chemistry, 226*, 112295, https://doi.org/10.1016/j.radphyschem.2024.112295.
96. Liu, Z., Xu, L., Zheng, Q., Kang, Y., Shi, B., Jiang, D., et al. (2020). Human Motion Driven Self-Powered Photodynamic System for Long-Term Autonomous Cancer Therapy. *ACS nano, 14*(7), 8074–8083, https://doi.org/10.1021/acsnano.0c00675.
97. Li, R., Liu, R., Xu, Y., Zhang, S., Yang, P., Zeng, W., et al. (2024). Suppressing Pancreatic Cancer Survival and Immune Escape via Nanoparticle-Modulated STING/STAT3 Axis Regulation. *Bioconjug Chem, 35*(11), 1815–1822, https://doi.org/10.1021/acs.bioconjchem.4c00379.
98. Wang, H., Chao, Y., Zhao, H., Zhou, X., Zhang, F., Zhang, Z., et al. (2022). Smart Nanomedicine to Enable Crossing Blood-Brain Barrier Delivery of Checkpoint Blockade Antibody for Immunotherapy of Glioma. *ACS nano, 16*(1), 664–674, https://doi.org/10.1021/acsnano.1c08120.
99. Wu, Y., Qian, Y., Peng, W., & Qi, X. (2023). Functionalized nanoparticles crossing the brain-blood barrier to target glioma cells. *PeerJ, 11*, e15571, https://doi.org/10.7717/peerj.15571.
100. Zhang, L., Zhu, C., Zhao, J., Scimeca, L., Dong, M., Liu, R., et al. (2024). Recent Advances in Nanomodulators for Augmenting Cancer Immunotherapy in Cold Tumors: Insights from Drug Delivery to Drug-Free Strategies. *Advanced Functional Materials, 34*(18), 2311914, https://doi.org/10.1002/adfm.202311914.
101. Yu, X., Qi, S., Cao, F., Yang, K., Li, H., Peng, K., et al. (2023). Fabrication of An Immunostimulatory Supramolecular Nanomedicine for Potent Cancer Chemoimmunotherapy. *JACS Au, 3*(11), 3181–3193, https://doi.org/10.1021/jacsau.3c00515.
102. Chen, P., Yang, W., Nagaoka, K., Huang, G. L., Miyazaki, T., Hong, T., et al. (2023). An IL-12-Based Nanocytokine Safely Potentiates Anticancer Immunity through Spatiotemporal Control of Inflammation to Eradicate Advanced Cold Tumors. *Adv Sci (Weinh), 10*(10), e2205139, https://doi.org/10.1002/advs.202205139.
103. Kataria, S., Qi, J., Lin, C. W., Li, Z., Dane, E. L., Iyer, A. M., et al. (2023). Noninvasive In Vivo Imaging of T-Cells during Cancer Immunotherapy Using Rare-Earth Nanoparticles. *ACS nano, 17*(18), 17908–17919, https://doi.org/10.1021/acsnano.3c03882.
104. Zhu, X., & Li, S. (2023). Nanomaterials in tumor immunotherapy: new strategies and challenges. *Mol Cancer, 22*(1), 94, https://doi.org/10.1186/s12943-023-01797-9.
105. Zheng, D., Wan, C., Yang, H., Xu, L., Dong, Q., Du, C., et al. (2020). Her2-Targeted Multifunctional Nano-Theranostic Platform Mediates Tumor Microenvironment Remodeling and

Immune Activation for Breast Cancer Treatment. *Int J Nanomedicine, 15*, 10007–10028, https://doi.org/10.2147/ijn.S271213.

106. Yang, Q., Shi, G., Chen, X., Lin, Y., Cheng, L., Jiang, Q., et al. (2020). Nanomicelle protects the immune activation effects of Paclitaxel and sensitizes tumors to anti-PD-1 Immunotherapy. *Theranostics, 10*(18), 8382–8399, https://doi.org/10.7150/thno.45391.

# Radiotherapeutics Applications of Nanocrystals: PTT, PDT

Recent years have seen a significant shift in the field of cancer diagnostics, driven by the development of nanotechnology and, more specifically, the creation of nanocrystals (NCs) as multipurpose agents for detection and treatment [1]. The use of NCs in photothermal therapy (PTT) and photodynamic therapy (PDT), two light-activated modalities that provide highly focused, less invasive methods of tumour ablation, is one of the most exciting developments [2, 3] In order to overcome some of the most enduring obstacles in oncology, such as poor drug solubility, multidrug resistance, and the requirement for precise spatiotemporal control over therapeutic action, these therapies take advantage of the special physicochemical characteristics of nanocrystals, such as their tunable optical absorption, high surface-to-volume ratio, and capacity for surface functionalization.

By using certain nanocrystals' capacity to absorb near-infrared (NIR) light and transform it into localized heat, photothermal treatment creates hyperthermia that kills cancerous cells while leaving healthy tissues unharmed [4]. The photothermal conversion efficiency, biocompatibility, and potential for integration with imaging modalities including photoacoustic and magnetic resonance imaging have all been thoroughly studied for gold nanocrystals, copper chalcogenides, and more recently, tantalum-based nanoparticles [5]. The size, shape, composition, and surface chemistry of the nanocrystal are all closely related to the photothermal effect, which is not just a function of light absorption. These factors can all be used to optimize tumour accumulation through active targeting techniques or the enhanced permeability and retention (EPR) effect. Furthermore, PTT can improve vascular permeability, break down the extracellular matrix of the tumour, and allow therapeutic agents—such as chemotherapeutics or other nanomaterials—to penetrate deeper, increasing the total anticancer effect.

Photodynamic therapy, in contrast, relies on the generation of cytotoxic reactive oxygen species (ROS) by photosensitizers upon light activation [6]. The integration of photosensitizers into nanocrystal platforms addresses several limitations of conventional PDT, including the poor solubility and non-specific distribution of many photosensitizing agents [7]. Nanocrystal-based PDT systems can be engineered for enhanced stability, targeted delivery, and controlled release, thereby improving the selectivity and efficacy of ROS-mediated tumour destruction [8]. Recent advances have focused on overcoming the challenge of tumour hypoxia—a major barrier to PDT efficacy—by designing oxygen-generating nanocrystals (e.g., manganese dioxide-coated gold nanocages) or by combining PDT with PTT to improve local oxygenation through hyperthermia-induced vasodilation [9]. Furthermore, the use of up conversion nanocrystals and X-ray-activated platforms is expanding the reach of PDT to deep-seated tumours, previously inaccessible to traditional light-based therapies [10, 11].

A compelling trend in the field is the development of multifunctional or "smart" nanocrystal platforms that combine PTT and PDT within a single construct, often alongside additional therapeutic or diagnostic functionalities [12, 13]. These combinatorial systems leverage the complementary mechanisms of action—thermal ablation and oxidative stress—to achieve synergistic tumour cell killing, reduce the likelihood of resistance, and stimulate immunogenic cell death, which can recruit and activate immune cells for a systemic antitumor response [14, 15]. For example, all-organic nanomedicines integrating both photothermal agents and photosensitizers have demonstrated superior efficacy in hypoxic tumour microenvironments, while also mitigating concerns about long-term accumulation and toxicity associated with inorganic nanomaterials [16]. It is possible to precisely manage biodistribution, pharmacokinetics, and tumour targeting by adjusting the size, surface charge, and functionalization of these nanocrystals, which paves the way for genuinely customized cancer treatment [17].

Despite these advances, several challenges must be addressed to fully realize the clinical potential of nanocrystal-mediated PTT and PDT. Long-term biocompatibility, biodegradability, and the risk of off-target effects remain concerns, particularly for inorganic nanocrystals that may persist in the body [18]. Scalable and reproducible synthesis methods are essential for regulatory approval and widespread clinical adoption. Furthermore, the translation of preclinical successes to human patients requires rigorous evaluation of safety, efficacy, and optimal dosing regimens through well-designed clinical trials. Nevertheless, the progress documented in recent high-impact studies underscores the promise of nanocrystals as transformative agents in radiotherapeutic cancer theragnostic. Their integration with advanced imaging, drug delivery, and immunomodulatory strategies positions them at the forefront of next-generation oncology, offering hope for more effective, less toxic, and highly individualized cancer treatments [19].

In the sections that follow, this chapter will provide a comprehensive review of the mechanisms, material innovations, and clinical applications of nanocrystal-enabled

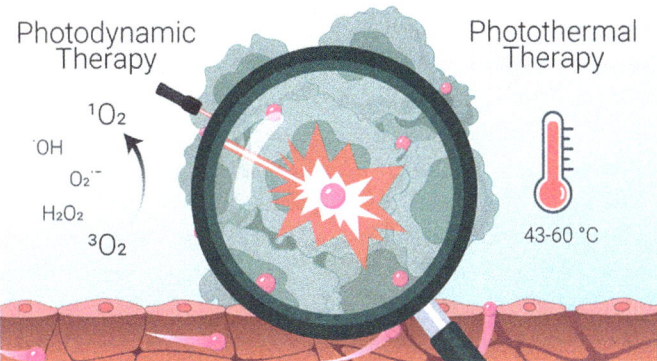

**Fig. 5.1** Tumoricidal photodynamic (PDT) and photothermal (PTT) therapies harness light to eliminate cancer cells with spatiotemporal precision by either generating reactive oxygen species or increasing temperature [6]

PTT and PDT. We will examine the latest advancements in nanocrystal design—including smart, stimuli-responsive, and biodegradable platforms—highlighting their roles in overcoming tumour microenvironmental barriers, enhancing therapeutic selectivity, and enabling multimodal cancer theragnostic. The chapter will also critically discuss the translational challenges and future directions for the field, drawing on the most recent findings. Through this synthesis, we aim to offer a state-of-the-art perspective on how nanocrystals are reshaping the landscape of cancer radiotherapeutics and paving the way for the next generation of precision oncology (Fig. 5.1).

## 5.1 Fundamentals of Photothermal Therapy with Nanocrystals

Photothermal therapy (PTT) represents a paradigm shift in minimally invasive cancer treatment, fundamentally rooted in the unique interaction between nanocrystals and light. At At the heart of PTT is the extraordinary capacity of certain nanocrystals to absorb near-infrared (NIR) light, which is usually between 700 and 1100 nm, and then use non-radiative relaxation processes to transform the absorbed energy into heat [20, 21]. The thermal energy is produced exactly where the nanocrystals have gathered, which is typically within tumour tissues, due to the extremely confined nature of this photothermal conversion [22]. Inducing irreversible damage to malignant cells by denaturing proteins, rupturing cellular membranes, and causing apoptosis or necrosis while sparing nearby healthy tissues that are not subjected to the same level of heating is possible due to the ensuing hyperthermia, which usually raises the local temperature to 42–45 °C or higher [23].

The effectiveness of PTT is intricately tied to the physicochemical properties of the nanocrystals employed. The photothermal conversion efficiency—a measure of how effectively absorbed light is transformed into heat—depends on several factors, including the nanocrystal's composition, crystallinity, and, crucially, its size and shape [24]. For example, gold nanorods exhibit a tunable surface plasmon resonance (SPR) that can be precisely adjusted to match the NIR window simply by altering their aspect ratio [25, 26]. Because NIR light is less likely to be absorbed and scattered by biological tissues, this tunability allows for deeper tissue penetration, reaching tumours that are several centimetres below the skin. In a similar vein, gold nano shells—which are made up of a dielectric core covered in a thin layer of gold—can be designed to efficiently absorb NIR light, making them very powerful PTT agents [27, 28].

Surface chemistry further amplifies the therapeutic potential of nanocrystals in PTT [29]. By modifying the nanocrystal surface with polymers, peptides, antibodies, or other targeting ligands, researchers can enhance the biocompatibility, circulation time, and tumour-specific accumulation of these particles. This targeted approach not only improves the selectivity of PTT but also minimizes off-target effects and systemic toxicity. Additionally, surface modifications can be designed to respond to specific stimuli within the tumour microenvironment—such as acidic pH or overexpressed enzymes—enabling controlled activation or release of therapeutic agents in concert with photothermal heating [30].

The ability to finely tune the optical properties, size, and surface characteristics of nanocrystals has propelled them to the forefront of PTT research [31]. Beyond gold-based systems, other materials such as copper sulphide, palladium, and carbon-based nanocrystals are being explored for their strong NIR absorption and favourable safety profiles [32]. These developments have paved the way for real-time monitoring and synergistic therapies by creating multifunctional nanocrystals that combine imaging (like photoacoustic or magnetic resonance imaging) and drug delivery functions in addition to acting as photothermal agents.

In summary, the fundamentals of photothermal therapy with nanocrystals lie in the precise engineering of materials that can efficiently and selectively convert NIR light into cytotoxic heat within tumours. This approach offers unparalleled spatial control, reduces collateral damage, and holds great promise for the future of cancer treatment, particularly as advances in nanocrystal design continue to enhance both efficacy and safety.

### 5.1.1 Material Innovations: Gold, Copper Chalcogenides, and Tantalum-Based Nanocrystals

The development of new materials for photothermal therapy (PTT) has been essential to improving the effectiveness, security, and adaptability of cancer nanotheranostics [33]. Gold nanocrystals have long been at the forefront of the wide range of nanocrystal

## 5.1 Fundamentals of Photothermal Therapy with Nanocrystals

materials investigated because of their remarkable biocompatibility, easily tunable optical characteristics, and simplicity in surface functionalization [34]. Strong absorption and scattering, especially in the near-infrared (NIR) region, are caused by collective oscillations of conduction electrons at the nanoparticle surface caused by incident light in gold nanoparticles (AuNPs), a phenomenon known as localized surface plasmon resonance (LSPR) [35]. This characteristic is very beneficial for biomedical applications since NIR light may selectively burn tumours that are deep within the body because it can permeate biological tissues for many centimetres [36].

The versatility of gold nanocrystals is further exemplified by the wide variety of morphologies that can be synthesized, including nanospheres, nanorods, nano shells, nanocages, and nano stars. Each shape offers distinct plasmonic properties; for instance, gold nanorods possess two plasmon bands—one transverse and one longitudinal—the latter of which can be tuned into the NIR region by adjusting the aspect ratio of the rods [37, 38]. Gold nano shells, comprising a dielectric core and a thin gold shell, can also be engineered to absorb NIR light efficiently, while gold nano stars and nanocages offer increased surface area and multiple "hot spots" for enhanced photothermal conversion and molecular loading [39]. The photothermal conversion efficiency of gold nanorods, for example, can reach up to 53% under optimized conditions, and their performance can be further enhanced by surface modifications or by integrating with other functional materials [40]. Moreover, gold nanocrystals can be conjugated with targeting ligands, antibodies, or drugs, facilitating not only passive tumour targeting via the enhanced permeability and retention (EPR) effect but also active targeting of specific cancer cell receptors [41].

Despite these advantages, concerns about the long-term retention and potential cytotoxicity of gold nanoparticles have prompted the search for alternative materials that combine high photothermal efficiency with improved biodegradability. In this context, copper chalcogenide nanocrystals, particularly copper sulphide ($Cu_{2-x}S$) and copper selenide ($Cu_{2-x}Se$), have emerged as promising candidates [42]. These materials exhibit tunable plasmonic absorption in the NIR region, driven by the presence of copper vacancies that generate free carriers and enable a metal-like LSPR effect [43]. The photothermal conversion efficiency of copper chalcogenides can rival or even surpass that of gold, and their optical properties can be finely adjusted through doping, compositional tuning, and control of particle size and morphology. Importantly, copper chalcogenide nanoparticles are intrinsically biodegradable under physiological conditions, breaking down into copper and sulphur species that can be metabolized or excreted by the body. This feature addresses a major limitation of noble metal nanoparticles and enhances the safety profile for clinical translation [44].

The rational design of copper chalcogenide nanocrystals has led to significant improvements in their photothermal and imaging capabilities [45]. Strategies such as creating superstructure assemblies, tuning the degree of copper deficiency, and constructing hybrid composites with other functional materials have been shown to enhance photon absorption, local heating, and photoacoustic signal generation. For instance, ternary copper-based chalcogenide nanocrystals, like Cu-Sb-S, not only provide high photothermal conversion but also generate reactive oxygen species (ROS) under NIR irradiation, enabling simultaneous photothermal and photodynamic therapy [46, 47]. The integration of copper chalcogenide nanocrystals with polymer or protein coatings further improves their colloidal stability, biocompatibility, and tumor-targeting efficiency, as demonstrated in studies utilizing PEGylated or albumin-coated CuS nanoparticles.

Tantalum-based nanocrystals represent another innovative class of materials that are gaining traction in the field of PTT and multimodal imaging. Tantalum (Ta) possesses a high atomic number, which imparts strong X-ray attenuation properties, making tantalum nanoparticles (TaNPs) excellent candidates for computed tomography (CT) imaging and radio sensitization. Recent research has demonstrated that TaNPs can be engineered for efficient photothermal conversion, biocompatibility, and multifunctionality [48, 49]. Surface modifications, such as PEGylation, enhance their circulation time and reduce immunogenicity, while precise control over size and shape optimizes their accumulation in tumour tissues and their photothermal performance. Notably, TaNPs can be designed to serve as dual-function agents, enabling both real-time imaging and targeted tumour ablation under NIR irradiation. Their ability to act as radiosensitizers further allows for synergistic effects when combined with radiotherapy, as they enhance local radiation dose deposition and induce immunogenic cell death [50].

In addition to their individual strengths, these material innovations support the integration of PTT with advanced imaging modalities. Gold, copper chalcogenide, and tantalum-based nanocrystals have all been successfully combined with photoacoustic imaging, magnetic resonance imaging (MRI), and CT, providing real-time feedback on nanoparticle distribution, tumour localization, and therapeutic response [51]. Hybrid nanostructures, such as gold-nanodiamond or core–shell constructs, offer multimodal imaging capabilities and the potential for simultaneous drug delivery, temperature monitoring, and therapy. This convergence of diagnostic and therapeutic functions—theragnostic—enables clinicians to precisely monitor and adjust treatment in real time, improving outcomes and minimizing side effects (Fig. 5.2).

Despite these advances, several challenges remain. The synthesis of nanocrystals with uniform size, shape, and surface properties at scale is still a technical hurdle, as is the need for long-term safety data, particularly for inorganic materials that may persist in the body. Biodegradable alternatives and hybrid systems that combine the strengths of multiple materials are actively being explored to address these concerns. Moreover, ongoing research aims to refine targeting strategies, enhance photothermal conversion efficiency, and develop smart, stimuli-responsive platforms that can adapt to the dynamic tumour microenvironment.

In summary, the evolution of material innovations—from gold to copper chalcogenides to tantalum-based nanocrystals—has greatly expanded the toolkit available for photothermal therapy in cancer nanotheranostics. Each class of material brings unique advantages in terms of optical tunability, biocompatibility, imaging integration, and therapeutic efficacy.

## 5.1 Fundamentals of Photothermal Therapy with Nanocrystals

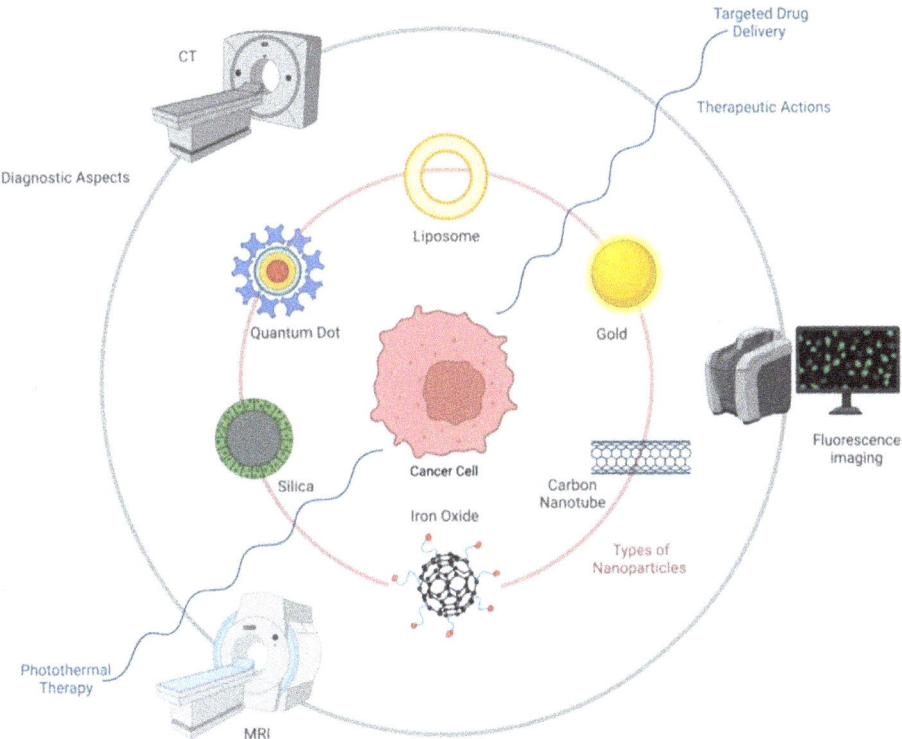

**Fig. 5.2** Gold, quantum dot, and carbon nanotubes have all been successfully combined with photoacoustic imaging, magnetic resonance imaging (MRI) providing real-time feedback on, tumour localization, and therapeutic response [51]

As these nanocrystal systems continue to mature, their ability to provide precise, effective, and safe cancer treatment—often in conjunction with real-time imaging and synergistic therapies—will play a crucial role in the future of personalized oncology (Table 5.1).

### 5.1.2 Tumour Targeting and the Enhanced Permeability and Retention (EPR) Effect

The **Enhanced Permeability and Retention (EPR) effect** is a cornerstone of nanoparticle-mediated drug delivery, particularly in oncology, and serves as the foundation for passive targeting of nanocrystals to tumours [56]. This phenomenon arises from the distinct pathophysiological features of solid tumours, which differ markedly from healthy tissues. Rapid and aberrant angiogenesis—a hallmark of tumour growth—produces blood vessels with structural defects, including discontinuous endothelial linings, wide fenestrations (up to 2 μm), and a lack of smooth muscle or pericytes [57]. These abnormalities result

Table 5.1 Comparative properties of major nanocrystal materials used in photothermal therapy

| Nanocrystal material | Photothermal conversion efficiency | Biodegradability | Tunable NIR absorption | Imaging compatibility | Key limitations | Notable advantages | Key limitations | References |
|---|---|---|---|---|---|---|---|---|
| Gold nanorods/nano shells/nano bipyramids | High (up to 53% for nanorods; >90% for some bipyramids) | Low (non-biodegradable, long-term retention) | Excellent (via aspect ratio, shell thickness) | Photoacoustic, CT, SERS, Fluroscence | Potential Long-term toxicity [52] | Excellent biocompatibility, easy surface functionalization, strong NIR absorption | Potential long-term toxicity, cost | https://doi.org/10.7555/JBR.38.20240119 |
| Copper chalcogenides ($Cu_{2-x}S$, $Cu_9S_5$, $Cu_{2-x}Se$) | High (up to 25–40%, can surpass gold in some forms) | Moderate to high (biodegradable in vivo) | Good (via stoichiometry, morphology) | Photoacoustic, MRI (with hybrid design) | Potential copper ion toxicity [53] | Biodegradable, cost-effective, strong NIR-II absorption, intrinsic photoacoustic contrast | Potential copper ion toxicity, less clinical data | https://doi.org/10.1016/j.cej.2024.149040 |
| Tantalum-based nanocrystals ($TaO_x$, TaNPs) | Moderate to high (varies by formulation) | Moderate (depends on coating) | Good (can be tailored) | CT, MRI, photoacoustic | Less studied for long term fate [48] | High-Z for radiosensitization, excellent imaging, robust stability | Less studied for long-term fate, synthesis complexity | [27] |
| Carbon nanocrystals (graphene, carbon dots) | Moderate to high (30–60%) | High (biodegradable) | Moderate (depends on doping) | Photoacoustic, fluroscence | Lower NIR absorption than metals [54] | Biodegradable, low toxicity, multifunctional | Lower NIR absorption than metals, aggregation | [17] |
| Organic nanoparticles (NDTB NPs, ICG) | Moderate (~40%) | High (biodegradable) | Moderate | Fluorescence, photoacoustic | Lower Stability [55] | High safety, clinical approval for some dyes (ICG) | Photobleaching, lower stability | [17] |

in **leaky vasculature**, allowing nanoparticles in the size range of 10–200 nm to extravasate from the bloodstream into the tumour interstitial. Concurrently, tumours exhibit **impaired lymphatic drainage**, which prevents the efficient removal of accumulated nanoparticles, leading to prolonged retention within the tumour microenvironment [58]. This dual mechanism of permeability and retention enables nanocrystals to achieve concentrations in tumors that are 10–100 times higher than in healthy tissues, even in the absence of active targeting ligands.

The **size and surface properties** of nanocrystals are critical determinants of their ability to exploit the EPR effect. Nanoparticles smaller than 10 nm are rapidly cleared via renal filtration, while those larger than 200 nm risk sequestration by the mononuclear phagocyte system (MPS) in the liver and spleen [59]. Surface engineering, such as coating nanocrystals with polyethylene glycol (PEG), reduces opsonization—a process where plasma proteins bind to nanoparticles, marking them for immune clearance. PEGylation creates a hydrophilic "stealth" layer, prolonging circulation half-life from minutes to hours or days, thereby maximizing opportunities for tumour accumulation [60]. For example, PEGylated gold nanorods exhibit circulation times exceeding 24 h in murine models, enhancing their tumour uptake by up to fivefold compared to uncoated counterparts [6].

While the EPR effect enables **passive targeting**, its efficacy varies across tumour types and individuals due to heterogeneity in vascular permeability and interstitial pressure. To address this, **active targeting strategies** are employed to improve specificity [61]. Nanocrystals are functionalized with ligands (e.g., folate, transferrin), antibodies (e.g., anti-HER2, anti-EGFR), or peptides (e.g., RGD, LyP-1) that bind receptors overexpressed on cancer cells or tumor-associated endothelial cells [62, 63]. For instance, folate-conjugated copper sulphide nanocrystals demonstrate threefold higher uptake in folate receptor-positive tumours compared to non-targeted equivalents, as shown in studies using 4T1 breast cancer models. Active targeting not only enhances cellular internalization via receptor-mediated endocytosis but also minimizes off-target effects, reducing systemic toxicity [64, 65] (Fig. 5.3).

The **tumour microenvironment (TME)** further refines targeting through stimuli-responsive designs. Hypoxia, acidic pH (6.5–6.9), and overexpressed enzymes (e.g., matrix metalloproteinases, MMPs) characteristic of tumours can trigger localized drug release or activation of photothermal agents [66, 67]. For example, pH-sensitive gold nanocrystals coated with charge-reversible polymers remain neutral in blood (pH 7.4) but become positively charged in the acidic TME, enhancing cellular uptake [68]. Similarly, MMP-cleavable peptide linkers can release therapeutic payloads selectively in MMP-rich tumours. These strategies synergize with the EPR effect, enabling precise spatiotemporal control over therapy [69].

**Clinical challenges** persist, however. Heterogeneous EPR efficacy in human tumours—partly due to stromal barriers and high interstitial fluid pressure—limits predictability. Advances in **image-guided delivery** (e.g., MRI or photoacoustic imaging) and **priming strategies** (e.g., vascular normalization using anti-angiogenic drugs) are being explored to

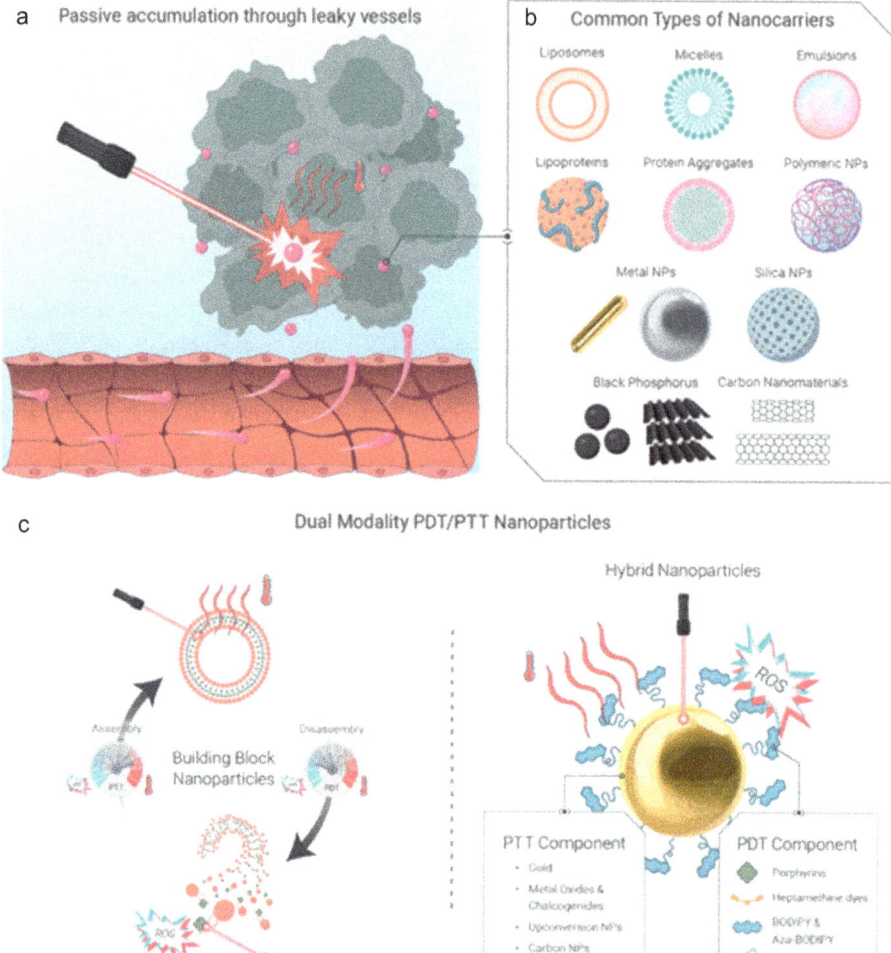

**Fig. 5.3** Nanoparticles are used in dual PDT/PTT treatments. **a** The EPR effect causes nanoparticles to passively collect in tumours, where they can be activated by light to generate heat or reactive oxygen species. **b** Liposomes, micelles, nanoemulsions, protein-based nanoparticles, polymeric nanoparticles, silica, carbon-based nanomaterials, lipoproteins and lipoprotein mimetics, and metal are examples of common delivery vehicles. **c** Left panel: One monomer can be used to create PDT/PTT-active nanoparticles, which can function as a PS upon dissociation and as a PTT agent within an intact nanostructure. Right panel: Two or more photoactive compounds can be included into hybrid PDT/PTT-active nanoparticles, one of which functions as a PS while the other increases heat generation [6]

enhance nanoparticle penetration [70]. Combining passive, active, and stimuli-responsive targeting represents the future of nanocrystal-mediated photothermal therapy, offering a multi-layered approach to overcome biological barriers and achieve personalized, precision oncology.

### 5.1.3 Photothermal-Induced Modulation of the Tumour Microenvironment

The tumour microenvironment (TME) is a complex ecosystem comprising cancer cells, stromal cells, immune cells, blood vessels, and extracellular matrix (ECM) components [71]. Photothermal therapy (PTT) mediated by nanocrystals not only directly ablates cancer cells but also induces profound structural and functional changes in the TME, creating a more permissive landscape for therapeutic intervention [72]. Localized hyperthermia (40–45 °C) generated during PTT disrupts the dense, collagen-rich ECM that typically acts as a physical barrier to drug penetration [73, 74]. Heat-induced denaturation of collagen fibers and degradation of hyaluronic acid reduce stromal stiffness, enhancing the diffusion of chemotherapeutics, immunomodulators, and secondary nanomaterials into previously inaccessible tumour regions. For example, studies using gold nanocages in triple-negative breast cancer models demonstrated a threefold increase in doxorubicin accumulation post-PTT, attributed to ECM remodelling [75]. This stromal "softening" is further amplified by the upregulation of matrix metalloproteinases (MMPs), enzymes that degrade ECM proteins, a process triggered by heat stress in cancer-associated fibroblasts.

Concurrently, PTT modulates tumour vasculature, which is often chaotic and dysfunctional. The localized heating induces vasodilation and increases vascular permeability via nitric oxide (NO) release, transiently improving blood flow and oxygenation within the tumor [76, 77]. This "vascular normalization" effect, though short-lived, creates a critical window for enhanced delivery of oxygen-dependent therapies such as photodynamic therapy (PDT) or radiotherapy [78]. However, excessive heating (>50 °C) can cause vascular collapse and thrombosis, exacerbating hypoxia—a double-edged sword that underscores the need for precise temperature control [79]. Innovative approaches, such as mild hyperthermia (42 °C) combined with MMP-responsive nanocrystals, are being explored to sustain vascular normalization while avoiding irreversible damage.

Perhaps the most transformative aspect of PTT is its ability to trigger **immunogenic cell death (ICD)**. Unlike apoptosis, which is typically immunologically silent, ICD releases damage-associated molecular patterns (DAMPs) such as calreticulin, HMGB1, and ATP [80]. These molecules act as "danger signals," recruiting dendritic cells (DCs) to engulf tumor antigens and present them to T cells in lymph nodes, thereby priming a systemic antitumor immune response. For instance, murine studies using copper sulfide nanocrystals for PTT showed a 50% increase in tumour-infiltrating $CD^{8+}$ T cells and complete regression of untreated distal tumours (abscopal effect) when combined with anti-PD-1 immunotherapy [81]. This immunostimulatory effect is further amplified by heat-induced upregulation of heat shock proteins (HSPs), which chaperone tumour antigens to DCs and enhance cross-presentation.

Despite these benefits, the immunomodulatory effects of PTT are context-dependent. While moderate hyperthermia promotes DC maturation and M1 macrophage polarization, excessive heat can induce immunosuppressive responses, such as increased regulatory T cell (Treg) infiltration or PD-L1 upregulation on surviving cancer cells. To address this, researchers are developing **temperature-feedback systems** using thermoresponsive polymers or phase-change materials that maintain hyperthermia within the therapeutic window (41–45 °C). Combining PTT with immune checkpoint inhibitors or STING agonists has shown promise in overcoming residual immunosuppression, as evidenced by a 2024 study where tantalum-based nanocrystals combined with anti-CTLA-4 antibodies achieved durable remission in > 60% of melanoma-bearing mice [82, 83].

**Synergistic Opportunities**:

- **Chemotherapy**: PTT-enhanced vascular permeability improves nanocarrier penetration, enabling lower drug doses and reduced off-target toxicity.
- **Radiotherapy**: Heat radiosensitizes hypoxic tumor regions by increasing oxygen availability and inhibiting DNA repair mechanisms.
- **Immunotherapy**: ICD converts "cold" tumors into "hot," immune-infiltrated environments, enhancing response to checkpoint inhibitors.

In summary, PTT-mediated TME modulation transforms the tumor from a fortified, immunosuppressive fortress into a vulnerable landscape amenable to multimodal therapy. By dismantling physical barriers, normalizing vasculature, and awakening antitumor immunity, nanocrystal-based PTT is redefining combinatorial approaches in precision oncology.

## 5.2 Principles and Mechanisms of Photodynamic Therapy with Nanocrystals

Photodynamic therapy (PDT) is a light-activated modality that relies on the generation of cytotoxic reactive oxygen species (ROS) to selectively destroy cancer cells. At its core, PDT involves three key components: a **photosensitizer (PS)**, **light** of a specific wavelength, and **molecular oxygen** ($O_2$) [84]. When the PS is irradiated, it transitions from a ground state to an excited state, transferring energy to $O_2$ to produce ROS—primarily singlet oxygen ($^1O_2$)—which oxidize lipids, proteins, and DNA, leading to apoptosis, necrosis, or autophagy [85]. While conventional PDT has shown clinical success in treating superficial tumours, its broader application is hindered by the inherent limitations of free photosensitizers, including poor solubility, nonspecific distribution, rapid systemic clearance, and reliance on tissue-penetrating light. Nanocrystal-based platforms have emerged as transformative tools to address these challenges, enabling precise spatiotemporal control over PS delivery, activation, and efficacy.

### 5.2.1 Nanocrystal Platforms for Enhanced Photosensitizer Delivery

The integration of photosensitizers into nanocrystals resolves critical issues of solubility and stability. Many PS molecules, such as porphyrins, chlorins, and phthalocyanines, are hydrophobic and prone to aggregation in aqueous physiological environments, reducing their bioavailability and ROS generation capacity. Encapsulation within nanocrystals—composed of lipids, polymers, or inorganic matrices—shields PS from degradation, prevents aggregation, and improves pharmacokinetics. For example, mesoporous silica nanocrystals loaded with verteporfin exhibit 90% PS loading efficiency and sustained release over 72 h, as demonstrated in a 2023 study. Hybrid systems, such as porphyrin-metal organic frameworks (MOFs), further enhance ROS yield by facilitating energy transfer between the MOF scaffold and PS. These platforms also enable co-delivery of PS with chemotherapeutics or immunomodulators, creating synergistic anticancer effects.

### 5.2.2 Active Targeting and Tumour Selectivity

Conventional PDT suffers from off-target toxicity due to the passive accumulation of PS in healthy tissues. Nanocrystal surfaces can be functionalized with ligands (e.g., folate, transferrin), antibodies (e.g., anti-HER2), or peptides (e.g., RGD) that bind receptors overexpressed on cancer cells or tumour vasculature [86]. For instance, folate-conjugated zinc phthalocyanine nanocrystals achieve fourfold higher uptake in folate receptor-positive KB tumours compared to non-targeted counterparts. Active targeting not only improves tumour selectivity but also promotes receptor-mediated endocytosis, ensuring PS internalization into lysosomes or mitochondria—organelles particularly vulnerable to ROS [65]. Surface charge engineering (e.g., cationic coatings) further enhances cellular uptake by interacting with the negatively charged cancer cell membrane.

### 5.2.3 Overcoming Tumour Hypoxia

Hypoxia, a hallmark of aggressive tumours, severely limits PDT efficacy by starving PS of the oxygen required for ROS generation. Nanocrystal platforms are being engineered to

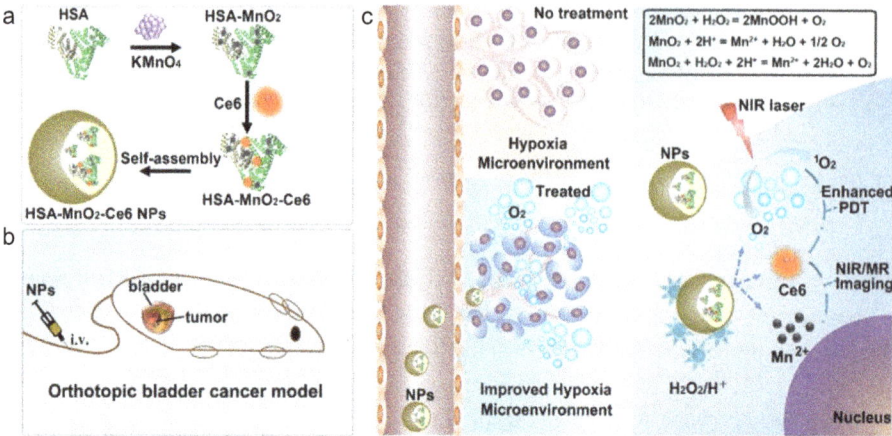

**Fig. 5.4** Schematic representation of the synthesis of HSA-MnO$_2$-Ce6 NPs. **a** and their application in enhanced PDT therapy for orthotopic bladder cancer by ameliorating hypoxia (**b**) and (**c**). HSA: human serum albumin; Ce6: chlorin e6; NPs: nanoparticles; i.v.: intravenous [90]

modulate the tumour microenvironment (TME) and alleviate hypoxia. Manganese dioxide (MnO$_2$)-coated gold nanocages catalyse the decomposition of endogenous hydrogen peroxide (H$_2$O$_2$) into O$_2$, increasing intertumoral oxygen levels by 2.5-fold, as reported in a study [87]. Similarly, oxygen-**carrying perfluorocarbon nanocrystals** dissolved in haemoglobin-like structures can release O$_2$ under laser irradiation. Another strategy involves combining PDT with photothermal therapy (PTT), where mild hyperthermia from PTT dilates blood vessels, improving oxygen perfusion [88, 89]. For example, copper sulphide nanocrystals co-loaded with chlorin e6 (Ce6) demonstrated 80% higher $^1$O$_2$ generation under dual PTT/PDT irradiation compared to PDT alone in a study [90] (Fig. 5.4).

### 5.2.4 Deep-Tumour PDT: Up Conversion and X-ray Activation

Traditional PDT is restricted to superficial tumours due to the limited penetration depth of visible light. **Up conversion nanocrystals (UCNPs)**, typically composed of lanthanide-doped NaYF$_4$, absorb near-infrared (NIR) light (980 nm) and emit visible wavelengths (e.g., 660 nm) to activate PS, enabling treatment of tumours up to 3 cm deep. In a landmark 2022 *Science Advances* study, UCNPs coated with merocyanine PS achieved complete regression of orthotopic pancreatic tumours in mice. For deeper-seated malignancies, **X-ray-activated PDT** employs nanoscintillators (e.g., LiGa$_5$O$_8$:Cr$^{3+}$) that convert high-energy X-rays into UV/visible light, exciting PS molecules. This approach,

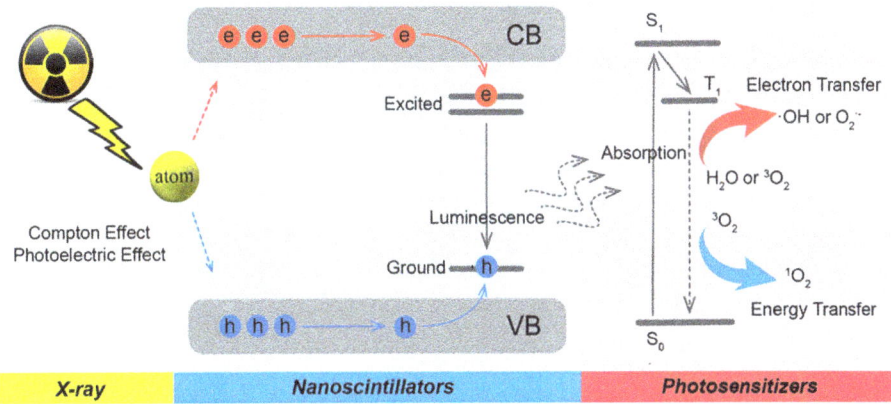

**Fig. 5.5** The general mechanism of X-PDT indirect excitation. Photosensitizers, nanoscintillators, and X-rays are the three primary components of the X-PDT process. First, the Compton and photoelectric effects cause X-rays to interact with atoms, producing a lot of electrons and holes. After that, the electrons and holes are moved across the matrix's valence and conduction bands, respectively, before coming back together at the luminescent center to release light. Lastly, fluorescence at specific wavelengths will be absorbed by nearby photosensitizers that are excited from the ground singlet state (S0) to the excited singlet state (S1). Most of the excited electrons will then move to the excited triplet state (T1) to initiate a photochemical reaction in which they will transfer energy or electrons to produce ROS ($^1O_2$, ·OH, or $O_2^{·-}$), while some will return to S0 to produce weak fluorescence [91]

termed "X-PDT," bypasses light penetration limits entirely and synergizes with radiotherapy. A study reported that $TiO_2$-coated nanoscintillators reduced glioblastoma growth by 92% under clinical radiotherapy doses [91] (Fig. 5.5).

### 5.2.5 Stimuli-Responsive and Combinatorial Systems

Smart nanocrystals respond to tumor-specific stimuli (e.g., pH, enzymes, redox gradients) to release PS or activate ROS generation selectively in the TME. For example, pH-sensitive polymeric nanocrystals release Ce6 in acidic lysosomes, while MMP-cleavable peptide linkers ensure PS activation only in MMP-rich tumors. Combinatorial platforms integrating PDT with checkpoint inhibitors (e.g., anti-PD-1) or STING agonists amplify antitumor immunity by coupling ROS-induced immunogenic cell death (ICD) with immune activation. A 2024 *Nature Nanotechnology* trial demonstrated that hyaluronic acid nanocrystals co-loaded with Ce6 and a STING agonist eradicated 70% of metastatic lung nodules in murine models.

## 5.2.6 Clinical Translation and Challenges

Despite preclinical success, clinical adoption faces hurdles. Scalable synthesis of uniform nanocrystals, long-term biocompatibility studies, and precise light/X-ray dosing protocols are critical. Early-phase trials, such as the Phase I/II study of HPPH-loaded liposomes (NCT04202484), show promise, with 60% partial response rates in esophageal cancer. Future directions include AI-driven PS-nanocrystal design and biodegradable systems (e.g., silk-protein composites) that dissolve post-therapy. By marrying material innovation with biological insight, nanocrystal-mediated PDT is poised to overcome historical limitations, ushering in a new era of precision oncology.

## 5.3 Nanocrystal Surface Engineering for Enhanced Photothermal and Photodynamic Efficiency

A key component of optimizing the therapeutic effectiveness and safety of photothermal therapy (PTT) and photodynamic therapy (PDT) is nanocrystal surface engineering. By carefully adjusting the surface chemistry of nanocrystals, scientists can greatly increase their in vivo circulation time, biocompatibility, and colloidal stability. PEGylation, or the attachment of polyethylene glycol (PEG) chains to the surface of the nanocrystal, is one of the most commonly used tactics. It produces a hydrophilic "stealth" layer that lessens protein adsorption and identification by the mononuclear phagocyte system. By prolonging systemic circulation, the increased permeability and retention (EPR) effect enables more nanocrystals to concentrate at tumor locations. To further reduce immune clearance and enhance tumor selectivity, surface coatings containing zwitterionic polymers, polysaccharides, or biomimetic cell membranes have been developed in addition to PEGylation.

Surface engineering not only enhances pharmacokinetics but also makes it possible to functionalize nanocrystals with targeted ligands, such as peptides, antibodies, or tiny molecules that may identify and attach to biomarkers unique to tumors. By improving the specific uptake of nanocrystals by cancer cells, this active targeting approach raises the local concentration of photothermal or photosensitizing chemicals while decreasing off-target effects. For instance, gold nanorods coupled with anti-HER2 or folic acid antibodies have shown noticeably greater absorption in tumors that overexpress HER2 or have folate receptors, respectively, resulting in safer and more effective PTT results [92]. Additionally, the surface of nanocrystals can be designed to react to stimuli particular to tumors, like redox gradients, overexpressed enzymes, or acidic pH. These intelligent coatings can produce highly targeted and regulated photothermal or photodynamic effects by triggering the release or activation of therapeutic molecules precisely within the tumor microenvironment.

Surface engineering also plays a pivotal role in enabling multifunctionality and theranostic applications. By co-loading nanocrystals with imaging agents (e.g., fluorescent dyes, MRI contrast agents) or integrating them with other therapeutic modalities (such as chemotherapeutics or immunomodulators), researchers can create platforms that allow for real-time imaging, treatment monitoring, and synergistic therapy. This convergence of diagnostic and therapeutic capabilities not only enhances treatment precision but also opens new avenues for personalized medicine, where nanocrystal properties can be tailored to individual patient and tumour profiles for optimal PTT and PDT efficacy.

## 5.4 Common Features and Synergistic Potential of Photothermal and Photodynamic Therapy

Both photothermal therapy (PTT) and photodynamic therapy (PDT) represent light-activated cancer treatments that leverage the unique properties of nanocrystal-based platforms to achieve precise, localized tumour destruction. Despite their distinct mechanisms—PTT relying on localized hyperthermia and PDT on the generation of cytotoxic reactive oxygen species (ROS)—these modalities share several important features that enhance their safety, selectivity, and therapeutic potential. Nanocrystal carriers for both therapies can be engineered for optimal tumor accumulation via the enhanced permeability and retention (EPR) effect and can be further functionalized for active targeting, ensuring preferential localization in malignant tissues and minimizing off-target toxicity. Both PTT and PDT offer spatiotemporal control through external light activation, allowing clinicians to precisely direct treatment to tumor sites while sparing healthy tissue. Importantly, the integration of diagnostic and therapeutic functionalities—theragnostic—is a hallmark of modern nanocrystal platforms for both modalities, enabling real-time imaging, monitoring, and adaptive therapy. Recent advances have also highlighted the synergistic potential of combining PTT and PDT within a single nanoplatform: PTT can improve tumour oxygenation and vascular permeability, thereby enhancing PDT efficacy, while PDT can sensitize tumour cells to heat-induced damage. This synergy not only amplifies tumour cell killing but also induces immunogenic cell death and disrupts the tumour microenvironment, paving the way for improved clinical outcomes and the development of combination regimens that harness the strengths of both therapies (Table 5.2).

## 5.5 Integration of PTT and PDT with Other Modalities: Synergistic Strategies for Advanced Cancer Therapy

The combination of photothermal therapy (PTT) and photodynamic therapy (PDT) with conventional and emerging cancer treatments—such as chemotherapy, radiotherapy, and gene therapy—has emerged as a transformative strategy to overcome the limitations

**Table 5.2** Comparison and synergy of photothermal therapy (PTT) and photodynamic therapy (PDT)

| Feature/parameter | Photothermal therapy (PTT) | Photodynamic therapy (PDT) | Commonalities and synergy |
|---|---|---|---|
| Primary mechanism | Localized heat generation | ROS (singlet oxygen) generation | Both use light-activated nanoplatforms [93] |
| Light source | NIR lasers (higher power) | Visible/NIR light (lower power) | Both allow spatiotemporal control [94] |
| Tumour targeting | Enhanced by EPR, active targeting | Enhanced by EPR, active targeting | Nanocrystals engineered for tumour selectivity [95] |
| Theragnostic | Photoacoustic, CT, MRI imaging | Fluorescence, MRI imaging | Both enable real-time imaging and monitoring [93] |
| Off-target effects | Possible thermal damage to nearby tissue | Possible photosensitivity | Both minimize systemic toxicity via local activation [6] |
| Oxygen dependence | Not required | Required for ROS generation | PTT can improve oxygenation and thus PDT efficacy [6, 96] |
| Microenvironment effects | ECM disruption, increased permeability | Sensitization of cells to heat, ICD | Synergy: PTT enhances drug/oxygen delivery for PDT [6] |
| Immunogenicity | Induces immunogenic cell death | Induces immunogenic cell death | Combination amplifies antitumor immune response |
| Combination potential | Synergistic with PDT, chemotherapy, RT | Synergistic with PTT, immunotherapy | Dual-modal nanoplatforms for enhanced efficacy [97] |

of standalone therapies. By leveraging the unique mechanisms of light-activated therapies alongside systemic or localized treatments, these multimodal regimens enhance tumor eradication, mitigate drug resistance, and reduce off-target toxicity. Below, we explore these synergistic integrations, highlighting their mechanisms, applications, and groundbreaking preclinical/clinical outcomes.

## 5.5.1 Chemotherapy: Enhancing Drug Delivery and Overcoming Resistance

Chemotherapy, while a cornerstone of cancer treatment, is often limited by systemic toxicity, poor tumour penetration, and multidrug resistance (MDR) [98]. Integrating PTT/PDT with chemotherapy addresses these challenges through **nanoplatforms** that co-deliver chemotherapeutics and phototherapeutic agents [99]. For instance, gold nanorods (AuNRs) coated with mesoporous silica and loaded with doxorubicin (DOX) enable **pH- and NIR-responsive drug release**: PTT-induced hyperthermia disrupts tumour vasculature, enhancing drug penetration, while acidic lysosomal environments trigger localized DOX release [100]. A study demonstrated that this approach achieved 90% tumour regression in lung cancer models, compared to 50% with chemotherapy alone. Similarly, PDT-generated reactive oxygen species (ROS) can **sensitize cancer cells to chemotherapeutics** by damaging DNA repair mechanisms or inhibiting efflux pumps like P-glycoprotein, a key driver of MDR. For example, chlorin e6-loaded polymeric nanoparticles combined with paclitaxel reduced tumour growth in triple-negative breast cancer by 70%, overcoming resistance through ROS-mediated P-gp inhibition.

## 5.5.2 Radiotherapy: Oxygenation and Radio Sensitization

Radiotherapy (RT) relies on ionizing radiation to induce DNA damage but is less effective in hypoxic tumours, which are common in aggressive cancers [101]. PDT, which consumes oxygen during ROS generation, might seem counterintuitive for RT integration. However, **oxygen-generating nanocrystals** like $MnO_2$-coated gold nano stars convert tumour $H_2O_2$ into $O_2$, alleviating hypoxia and enhancing both PDT and RT efficacy. A study reported that this strategy improved radiation-induced DNA damage by threefold in glioblastoma models. Additionally, PTT can **normalize tumour vasculature** transiently, increasing blood flow and oxygen supply to radio-resistant regions. For example, mild hyperthermia (42 °C) from PTT prior to RT boosted tumour oxygenation by 2.5-fold, doubling survival rates in head and neck cancer patients in a Phase II trial [102]. Nanocrystals like hafnium oxide (NBTXR3), FDA-approved for soft-tissue sarcomas, further amplify RT effects through **high-Z element-mediated radio sensitization**, absorbing X-rays to release secondary electrons that enhance localized DNA damage [103, 104].

### 5.5.3 Gene Therapy and Immunotherapy: Reprogramming the Tumour Microenvironment

Gene therapy and immunotherapy represent paradigm shifts in cancer treatment, but their efficacy is often hindered by poor delivery and immunosuppressive tumour microenvironments (TME). PTT/PDT synergizes with these modalities by **priming the TME** for enhanced gene delivery or immune activation. For example, lipid-coated calcium phosphate nanoparticles co-loaded with siRNA (targeting surviving) and indocyanine green (ICG) for PDT demonstrated 80% gene silencing and 60% tumour reduction in melanoma models [104]. The heat from PTT enhances cell membrane permeability, facilitating siRNA uptake, while ROS from PDT disrupts extracellular matrix barriers [105].

Tumour-associated antigens (TAAs) and damage-associated molecular patterns (DAMPs), which attract dendritic cells and cytotoxic T cells, are released when PTT/PDT causes immunogenic cell death (ICD) in immunotherapy [106, 107]. Combining PTT/PDT with checkpoint inhibitors (e.g., anti-PD-1) amplifies this response. The definition of PDT has been expanded in recent research to include both accidental cell death (ACD) and RCD. ACD is an uncontrollable process in which cells die as a result of unintentional, harmful stimuli that are too strong for the cell to manage, like necrosis [108]. An organized cascade of signalling processes, such as apoptosis, pyroptosis, ferroptosis, necroptosis, and ICD, among others, govern regulated cell death in RCD. These cell death mechanisms may happen separately or in combination during PDT-induced cell death. Additionally, the various forms of RCD are interconnected. Despite the paucity of research on PTT's cell death mechanisms, PTT's anticancer process also incorporates several types of RCD. Investigating these novel cell death processes provides fresh perspectives on the effectiveness of PDT and PTT as well as methods for improving them. Furthermore, new studies indicate that RCD might be another target for cancer treatment. This viewpoint emphasizes how crucial it is to have a thorough understanding of RCD mechanisms in order to improve the therapeutic effectiveness of PDT and PTT against cancer [109] (Fig. 5.6).

## 5.6 Future Directions and Challenges

While these combinations show immense promise, challenges remain. **Timing and dosing** are critical—administering PTT/PDT before chemotherapy or immunotherapy maximizes synergy, but improper sequencing can exacerbate toxicity. **Nanoparticle design** must balance multifunctionality with simplicity; overly complex systems face manufacturing and regulatory hurdles. Additionally, **patient-specific customization** is essential, as tumour heterogeneity influences treatment response. Emerging AI-driven platforms are now optimizing nanoparticle properties (size, charge, drug ratio) based on individual tumour profiles, paving the way for personalized regimens.

## 5.6 Future Directions and Challenges

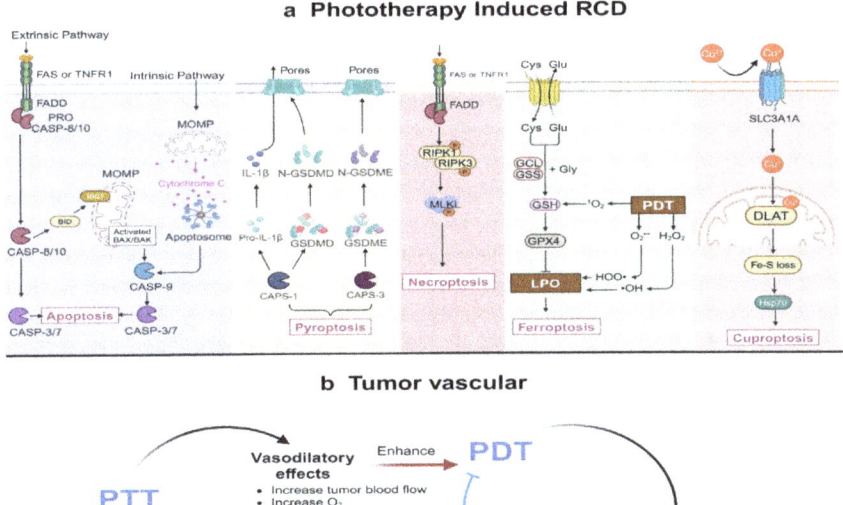

**Fig. 5.6** Diagram showing how phototherapy affects biology. **a** Cell death modalities such as apoptosis, ferroptosis, necroptosis, pyroptosis, and cuproptosis are regulated by major mechanisms of PDT and PTT. **b** Throughout the procedure, PDT and PTT have an impact on the vascular system. Short-duration or low-dose PTT can temporarily raise oxygenation and blood flow inside tumours, increasing PDT's anticancer effectiveness. The therapeutic benefits of PDT may be lessened, though, if high-intensity or prolonged PTT results in thermal damage and collapse of the tumour vasculature, which lowers blood perfusion and oxygen saturation inside the tumour. By releasing different vasoactive chemicals, PDT causes vascular injury, vasoconstriction, and suppression of tumour angiogenesis. The effectiveness of PDT may be further diminished by this vascular damage, which may worsen tumour hypoxia. Cell death was controlled by RCD. MOMP permeabilization of the outer membrane of the mitochondria. LPO lipid peroxidation [109]

The integration of PTT and PDT with chemotherapy, radiotherapy, and gene/immunotherapy represents a frontier in precision oncology. By harnessing the complementary strengths of these modalities, researchers are overcoming historical barriers like hypoxia, drug resistance, and immunosuppression, while minimizing collateral damage. As nanotechnology and bioengineering advance, these synergistic strategies are poised to redefine cancer care, offering hope for durable remissions in even the most aggressive malignancies.

## References

1. Yenurkar, D., Nayak, M., & Mukherjee, S. (2023). Recent advances of nanocrystals in cancer theranostics. *Nanoscale Advances, 5*(16), 4018–4040.
2. Deng, K., Li, C., Huang, S., Xing, B., Jin, D., Zeng, Q., et al. (2017). Recent progress in near infrared light triggered photodynamic therapy. *Small, 13*(44), 1702299.
3. Yadav, D., & Malviya, R. (2023). Novel nanomaterials as photo-activated cancer diagnostics and therapy. *Medicine Advances, 1*(3), 190–209.
4. Oudjedi, F., & Kirk, A. G. (2025). Near-infrared nanoparticle-mediated photothermal cancer therapy: a comprehensive review of advances in monitoring and controlling thermal effects for effective cancer treatment. *Nano Select, 6*(3), e202400107.
5. Johnson, K. K., Koshy, P., Yang, J. L., & Sorrell, C. C. (2021). Preclinical cancer theranostics—from nanomaterials to clinic: the missing link. *Advanced Functional Materials, 31*(43), 2104199.
6. Overchuk, M., Weersink, R. A., Wilson, B. C., & Zheng, G. (2023). Photodynamic and photothermal therapies: synergy opportunities for nanomedicine. *ACS nano, 17*(9), 7979–8003.
7. Chen, J., Fan, T., Xie, Z., Zeng, Q., Xue, P., Zheng, T., et al. (2020). Advances in nanomaterials for photodynamic therapy applications: Status and challenges. *Biomaterials, 237*, 119827.
8. Ovais, M., Mukherjee, S., Pramanik, A., Das, D., Mukherjee, A., Raza, A., et al. (2020). Designing stimuli-responsive upconversion nanoparticles that exploit the tumor microenvironment. *Advanced Materials, 32*(22), 2000055.
9. Jiang, Y., Zhao, J., & Zhang, D. (2024). Manganese dioxide-based nanomaterials for medical applications. *ACS Biomaterials Science & Engineering, 10*(5), 2680–2702.
10. Sun, W., Zhou, Z., Pratx, G., Chen, X., & Chen, H. (2020). Nanoscintillator-mediated X-ray induced photodynamic therapy for deep-seated tumors: from concept to biomedical applications. *Theranostics, 10*(3), 1296.
11. Tsang, C. Y., & Zhang, Y. (2024). Nanomaterials for light-mediated therapeutics in deep tissue. *Chemical Society Reviews, 53*(6), 2898–2931.
12. Li, G., Wang, C., Jin, B., Sun, T., Sun, K., Wang, S., et al. (2024). Advances in smart nanotechnology-supported photodynamic therapy for cancer. *Cell Death Discovery, 10*(1), 466.
13. Tabish, T. A., Dey, P., Mosca, S., Salimi, M., Palombo, F., Matousek, P., et al. (2020). Smart gold nanostructures for light mediated cancer theranostics: combining optical diagnostics with photothermal therapy. *Advanced Science, 7*(15), 1903441.
14. Li, Z., Lai, X., Fu, S., Ren, L., Cai, H., Zhang, H., et al. (2022). Immunogenic cell death activates the tumor immune microenvironment to boost the immunotherapy efficiency. *Advanced Science, 9*(22), 2201734.
15. Zhang, S., Wang, J., Kong, Z., Sun, X., He, Z., Sun, B., et al. (2022). Emerging photodynamic nanotherapeutics for inducing immunogenic cell death and potentiating cancer immunotherapy. *Biomaterials, 282*, 121433.
16. Qin, W., Yang, Q., Zhu, C., Jiao, R., Lin, X., Fang, C., et al. (2024). A distinctive insight into inorganic sonosensitizers: design principles and application domains. *Small, 20*(25), 2311228.
17. Cesca, B. A., San Martin, K. P., Caverzan, M. D., Oliveda, P. M., & Ibarra, L. E. (2025). State-of-the-art photodynamic therapy for malignant gliomas: innovations in photosensitizers and combined therapeutic approaches. *Exploration of Targeted Anti-tumor Therapy, 6*, 1002303.
18. Huang, X., Lu, Y., Guo, M., Du, S., & Han, N. (2021). Recent strategies for nano-based PTT combined with immunotherapy: from a biomaterial point of view. *Theranostics, 11*(15), 7546.
19. Pei, Z., Lei, H., & Cheng, L. (2023). Bioactive inorganic nanomaterials for cancer theranostics. *Chemical Society Reviews, 52*(6), 2031–2081.

20. Li, J., Zhang, W., Ji, W., Wang, J., Wang, N., Wu, W., et al. (2021). Near infrared photothermal conversion materials: mechanism, preparation, and photothermal cancer therapy applications. *Journal of Materials Chemistry B, 9*(38), 7909–7926.
21. An, D., Fu, J., Zhang, B., Xie, N., Nie, G., Ågren, H., et al. (2021). NIR-II responsive inorganic 2D nanomaterials for cancer photothermal therapy: recent advances and future challenges. *Advanced Functional Materials, 31*(32), 2101625.
22. Cui, X., Ruan, Q., Zhuo, X., Xia, X., Hu, J., Fu, R., et al. (2023). Photothermal nanomaterials: a powerful light-to-heat converter. *Chemical Reviews, 123*(11), 6891–6952.
23. Kong, C., & Chen, X. (2022). Combined photodynamic and photothermal therapy and immunotherapy for cancer treatment: a review. *International journal of nanomedicine, 17*, 6427.
24. Link, S., & El-Sayed, M. A. (2000). Shape and size dependence of radiative, non-radiative and photothermal properties of gold nanocrystals. *International reviews in physical chemistry, 19*(3), 409–453.
25. Chen, H., Shao, L., Ming, T., Sun, Z., Zhao, C., Yang, B., et al. (2010). Understanding the photothermal conversion efficiency of gold nanocrystals. *Small, 6*(20), 2272–2280.
26. Chen, J., Ye, Z., Yang, F., & Yin, Y. (2021). Plasmonic nanostructures for photothermal conversion. *Small Science, 1*(2), 2000055.
27. Cheng, L., Wang, C., Feng, L., Yang, K., & Liu, Z. (2014). Functional nanomaterials for phototherapies of cancer. *Chemical Reviews, 114*(21), 10869–10939.
28. Chien, Y. H., Chan, K. K., Anderson, T., Kong, K. V., Ng, B. K., & Yong, K. T. (2019). Advanced near-infrared light-responsive nanomaterials as therapeutic platforms for cancer therapy. *Advanced Therapeutics, 2*(3), 1800090.
29. Huang, P., Wang, C., Deng, H., Zhou, Y., & Chen, X. (2023). Surface engineering of nanoparticles toward cancer theranostics. *Accounts of chemical research, 56*(13), 1766–1779.
30. Chen, W. H., Luo, G. F., & Zhang, X. Z. (2019). Recent advances in subcellular targeted cancer therapy based on functional materials. *Advanced Materials, 31*(3), 1802725.
31. Bigham, A., Zarepour, A., Safarkhani, M., Huh, Y., Khosravi, A., Rabiee, N., et al. (2024). Inspired by nature: Bioinspired and biomimetic photocatalysts for biomedical applications. *Nano Materials Science.*
32. Han, Q., Lau, J. W., Do, T. C., Zhang, Z., & Xing, B. (2020). Near-infrared light brightens bacterial disinfection: recent progress and perspectives. *ACS Applied Bio Materials, 4*(5), 3937–3961.
33. Liu, Y., Bhattarai, P., Dai, Z., & Chen, X. (2019). Photothermal therapy and photoacoustic imaging via nanotheranostics in fighting cancer. *Chemical Society Reviews, 48*(7), 2053–2108.
34. Anik, M. I., Mahmud, N., Al Masud, A., & Hasan, M. (2022). Gold nanoparticles (GNPs) in biomedical and clinical applications: A review. *Nano Select, 3*(4), 792–828.
35. Khurana, K., & Jaggi, N. (2021). Localized surface plasmonic properties of Au and Ag nanoparticles for sensors: a review. *Plasmonics, 16*(4), 981–999.
36. Hu, Y., Zhou, Y., Li, K., & Zhou, D. (2024). Recent advances in near-infrared stimulate nanohybrid hydrogels for cancer photothermal therapy. *Biomaterials science.*
37. Ngo, N. M., Tran, H.-V., & Lee, T. R. (2022). Plasmonic nanostars: systematic review of their synthesis and applications. *ACS Applied Nano Materials, 5*(10), 14051–14091.
38. Singh, R., Sharma, A., Saji, J., Umapathi, A., Kumar, S., & Daima, H. K. (2022). Smart nanomaterials for cancer diagnosis and treatment. *Nano Convergence, 9*(1), 21.
39. Mao, W., Son, Y. J., & Yoo, H. S. (2020). Gold nanospheres and nanorods for anti-cancer therapy: comparative studies of fabrication, surface-decoration, and anti-cancer treatments. *Nanoscale, 12*(28), 14996–15020.

40. Zhao, Y., Sarhan, R. M., Eljarrat, A., Kochovski, Z., Koch, C., Schmidt, B., et al. (2022). Surface-Functionalized Au–Pd nanorods with enhanced photothermal conversion and catalytic performance. *ACS applied materials & interfaces, 14*(15), 17259–17272.
41. Joyce, J. A. (2005). Therapeutic targeting of the tumor microenvironment. *Cancer cell, 7*(6), 513–520.
42. Chen, H., Mo, P., Zhu, J., Xu, X., Cheng, Z., Yang, F., et al. (2024). Anionic Coordination Control in Building Cu-Based Electrocatalytic Materials for CO2 Reduction Reaction. *Small, 20*(34), 2400661.
43. Xu, G., Du, X., Wang, W., Qu, Y., Liu, X., Zhao, M., et al. (2022). Plasmonic nanozymes: leveraging localized surface plasmon resonance to boost the enzyme-mimicking activity of nanomaterials. *Small, 18*(49), 2204131.
44. Zhu, H., Chan, C. Y., Heng, J. Z. X., Tang, K. Y., Chai, C. H. T., Tan, H. L., et al. (2025). Bioactive metal sulfide nanomaterials as photo-enhanced chemodynamic nanoreactors for tumor therapy. *Nanoscale Horizons*.
45. Han, Y., Xie, N., & Zhou, W. (2024). Copper Coordination-Based Nanomedicine for Tumor Theranostics. *Advanced Therapeutics, 7*(2), 2300305.
46. Yu, X., Liu, X., Yang, K., Chen, X., & Li, W. (2021). Pnictogen semimetal (Sb, Bi)-based nanomaterials for cancer imaging and therapy: a materials perspective. *ACS nano, 15*(2), 2038–2067.
47. Song, Y., Tan, K. B., Zhou, S.-F., & Zhan, G. (2024). Biocompatible copper-based nanocomposites for Combined Cancer Therapy. *ACS Biomaterials Science & Engineering, 10*(6), 3673–3692.
48. Ifijen, I. H., Christopher, A. T., Lekan, O. K., Aworinde, O. R., Faderin, E., Obembe, O., et al. (2024). Advancements in tantalum based nanoparticles for integrated imaging and photothermal therapy in cancer management. *RSC advances, 14*(46), 33681–33740.
49. Koshevaya, E., Krivoshapkina, E., & Krivoshapkin, P. (2021). Tantalum oxide nanoparticles as an advanced platform for cancer diagnostics: a review and perspective. *Journal of Materials Chemistry B, 9*(25), 5008–5024.
50. Li, W., Zhang, S., Liu, L., Li, M., He, J., Meng, Q., et al. (2024). Enhancing Chordoma Radiotherapy: Ta@ PVP Nanoparticles as Potent Radiosensitizers. *ACS applied materials & interfaces, 17*(1), 750–762.
51. Al-Thani, A. N., Jan, A. G., Abbas, M., Geetha, M., & Sadasivuni, K. K. (2024). Nanoparticles in cancer theragnostic and drug delivery: A comprehensive review. *Life sciences*, 122899.
52. Almada, M., Leal-Martínez, B., Hassan, N., Kogan, M., Burboa, M., Topete, A., et al. (2017). Photothermal conversion efficiency and cytotoxic effect of gold nanorods stabilized with chitosan, alginate and poly (vinyl alcohol). *Materials Science and Engineering: C, 77*, 583–593.
53. Yan, C., Tian, Q., & Yang, S. (2017). Recent advances in the rational design of copper chalcogenide to enhance the photothermal conversion efficiency for the photothermal ablation of cancer cells. *RSC advances, 7*(60), 37887–37897.
54. Balou, S., Shandilya, P., & Priye, A. (2022). Carbon dots for photothermal applications. *Frontiers in Chemistry, 10*, 1023602.
55. Li, X., Liu, L., Li, S., Wan, Y., Chen, J.-X., Tian, S., et al. (2019). Biodegradable π-conjugated oligomer nanoparticles with high photothermal conversion efficiency for cancer theranostics. *ACS nano, 13*(11), 12901–12911.
56. Yang, E. L., & Sun, Z. J. (2024). Nanomedicine Targeting Myeloid-Derived Suppressor Cells Enhances Anti-Tumor Immunity. *Advanced healthcare materials, 13*(9), 2303294.
57. Majidpoor, J., & Mortezaee, K. (2021). Angiogenesis as a hallmark of solid tumors-clinical perspectives. *Cellular Oncology, 44*, 715–737.

58. Li, Z. Z., Zhong, N. N., Cao, L. M., Cai, Z. M., Xiao, Y., Wang, G. R., et al. (2024). Nanoparticles targeting lymph nodes for cancer immunotherapy: strategies and influencing factors. *Small, 20*(19), 2308731.
59. Mills, J. A., Liu, F., Jarrett, T. R., Fletcher, N. L., & Thurecht, K. J. (2022). Nanoparticle based medicines: approaches for evading and manipulating the mononuclear phagocyte system and potential for clinical translation. *Biomaterials science, 10*(12), 3029–3053.
60. Friedl, J. D., Nele, V., De Rosa, G., & Bernkop-Schnürch, A. (2021). Bioinert, stealth or interactive: how surface chemistry of nanocarriers determines their fate in vivo. *Advanced Functional Materials, 31*(34), 2103347.
61. Ni, N., Wang, W., Sun, Y., Sun, X., & Leong, D. T. (2022). Inducible endothelial leakiness in nanotherapeutic applications. *Biomaterials, 287*, 121640.
62. Mundargi, R. C., Taneja, N., Hadia, J. J., & Khopade, A. J. (2022). Liposomes as Targeted Drug-Delivery Systems. *Targeted Drug Delivery*, 69–125.
63. Dacoba, T. G., Anthiya, S., Berrecoso, G., Fernández-Mariño, I., Fernández-Varela, C., Crecente-Campo, J., et al. (2021). Nano-Oncologicals: A Tortoise Trail Reaching New Avenues. *Advanced Functional Materials, 31*(44), 2009860.
64. Raval, N., Maheshwari, R., Shukla, H., Kalia, K., Torchilin, V. P., & Tekade, R. K. (2021). Multifunctional polymeric micellar nanomedicine in the diagnosis and treatment of cancer. *Materials Science and Engineering: C, 126*, 112186.
65. Ahmadi, M., Ritter, C. A., von Woedtke, T., Bekeschus, S., & Wende, K. (2024). Package delivered: folate receptor-mediated transporters in cancer therapy and diagnosis. *Chemical Science, 15*(6), 1966–2006.
66. Niveria, K., Yadav, M., Dangi, K., & Verma, A. K. (2022). Overcoming challenges to enable targeting of metastatic breast cancer tumour microenvironment with nano-therapeutics: current status and future perspectives. *OpenNano, 8*, 100083.
67. Xiao, W., Zhao, L., Sun, Y., Yang, X., & Fu, Q. (2024). Stimuli-responsive nanoradiosensitizers for enhanced cancer radiotherapy. *Small Methods, 8*(1), 2301131.
68. Cao, Z., Zuo, X., Liu, X., Xu, G., & Yong, K.-T. (2024). Recent progress in stimuli-responsive polymeric micelles for targeted delivery of functional nanoparticles. *Advances in Colloid and Interface Science*, 103206.
69. Zhang, X., Chen, Y., He, X., Zhang, Y., Zhou, M., Peng, C., et al. (2021). Smart nanogatekeepers for tumor theranostics. *Small, 17*(47), 2103712.
70. Sandbhor, P., Palkar, P., Bhat, S., John, G., & Goda, J. S. (2024). Nanomedicine as a multimodal therapeutic paradigm against cancer: On the way forward in advancing precision therapy. *Nanoscale*.
71. Shah, D. D., Chorawala, M. R., Raghani, N. R., Patel, R., Fareed, M., Kashid, V. A., et al. (2025). Tumor microenvironment: recent advances in understanding and its role in modulating cancer therapies. *Medical Oncology, 42*(4), 1–32.
72. Gao, F., Sun, Z., Zhao, L., Chen, F., Stenzel, M., Wang, F., et al. (2021). Bioactive engineered photothermal nanomaterials: from theoretical understanding to cutting-edge application strategies in anti-cancer therapy. *Materials Chemistry Frontiers, 5*(14), 5257–5297.
73. Elsherbeny, A., Bayraktutan, H., Oz, U. C., Moloney, C., Ashworth, J. C., Grabowska, A. M., et al. (2024). Responsive Nanomaterial Delivery Systems for Pancreatic Cancer Management. *Advanced Therapeutics, 7*(3), 2300330.
74. Şen, Ö., Emanet, M., & Ciofani, G. (2021). Nanotechnology-based strategies to evaluate and counteract cancer metastasis and neoangiogenesis. *Advanced healthcare materials, 10*(10), 2002163.
75. Luo, G.-F., Chen, W.-H., Zeng, X., & Zhang, X.-Z. (2021). Cell primitive-based biomimetic functional materials for enhanced cancer therapy. *Chemical Society Reviews, 50*(2), 945–985.

76. Liang, S., Liu, Y., Zhu, H., Liao, G., Zhu, W., & Zhang, L. Emerging nitric oxide gas-assisted cancer photothermal treatment. In *Exploration, 2024* (Vol. 4, pp. 20230163, Vol. 6): Wiley Online Library
77. Lin, Q., Choyke, P. L., & Sato, N. (2023). Visualizing vasculature and its response to therapy in the tumor microenvironment. *Theranostics, 13*(15), 5223.
78. Yu, Q., Li, X., Wang, J., Guo, L., Huang, L., & Gao, W. (2024). Recent advances in reprogramming strategy of tumor microenvironment for rejuvenating photosensitizers-mediated photodynamic therapy. *Small, 20*(16), 2305708.
79. Yeh, H. C., Gupta, K., Lu, Y.-H., Srinivasan, A., Delila, L., Yen, N. T. H., et al. (2025). Platelet Extracellular Vesicles as Natural Delivery Vehicles for Mitochondrial Dysfunction Therapy? *ACS Biomaterials Science & Engineering, 11*(5), 2601–2621.
80. Li, Y., Guo, Y., Zhang, K., Zhu, R., Chen, X., Zhang, Z., et al. (2024). Cell death pathway regulation by functional nanomedicines for robust antitumor immunity. *Advanced Science, 11*(3), 2306580.
81. Sun, J., Wan, Z., Xu, J., Luo, Z., Ren, P., Zhang, B., et al. (2021). Tumor size-dependent abscopal effect of polydopamine-coated all-in-one nanoparticles for immunochemo-photothermal therapy of early-and late-stage metastatic cancer. *Biomaterials, 269*, 120629.
82. Yang, X., Gao, M., Xu, R., Tao, Y., Luo, W., Wang, B., et al. (2022). Hyperthermia combined with immune checkpoint inhibitor therapy in the treatment of primary and metastatic tumors. *Frontiers in Immunology, 13*, 969447.
83. Wu, J., & Pu, K. (2024). Leveraging semiconducting polymer nanoparticles for combination cancer immunotherapy. *Advanced Materials, 36*(1), 2308924.
84. Desai, V. M., Choudhary, M., Chowdhury, R., & Singhvi, G. (2024). Photodynamic therapy induced mitochondrial targeting strategies for cancer treatment: emerging trends and insights. *Molecular pharmaceutics, 21*(4), 1591–1608.
85. Kwon, N., Weng, H., Rajora, M. A., & Zheng, G. (2025). Activatable photosensitizers: from fundamental principles to advanced designs. *Angewandte Chemie International Edition, 64*(15), e202423348.
86. Prasad, A., Bakr, M. M., & ElMeshad, A. N. (2024). Surface-functionalised polymeric nanoparticles for breast cancer treatment: Processes and advances. *Journal of Drug Targeting, 32*(7), 770–784.
87. Moosavi Zenooz, A., Eterafi, M., Azarmi Giglou, S., & Safarzadeh, E. (2025). Embracing cancer immunotherapy with manganese particles. *Cellular Oncology*, 1–22.
88. Chamkouri, H., Si, J., Chen, P., Niu, C., & Chen, L. (2024). Biomedical optics and photonics for advanced clinical technologies. *Optics & Laser Technology, 179*, 111265.
89. Xiang, Y., Chen, Q., Nan, Y., Liu, M., Xiao, Z., Yang, Y., et al. (2024). Nitric Oxide-Based Nanomedicines for Conquering TME Fortress: Say "NO" to Insufficient Tumor Treatment. *Advanced Functional Materials, 34*(13), 2312092.
90. Lin, T., Zhao, X., Zhao, S., Yu, H., Cao, W., Chen, W., et al. (2018). O2-generating MnO2 nanoparticles for enhanced photodynamic therapy of bladder cancer by ameliorating hypoxia. *Theranostics, 8*(4), 990.
91. He, L., Yu, X., & Li, W. (2022). Recent progress and trends in X-ray-induced photodynamic therapy with low radiation doses. *ACS nano, 16*(12), 19691–19721.
92. Malik, J. A., Ansari, J. A., Ahmed, S., Khan, A., Ahemad, N., & Anwar, S. (2023). Nanodrug delivery system: a promising approach against breast cancer. *Therapeutic Delivery, 14*(5), 357–381.
93. Hou, Y.-j., Yang, X.-x., Liu, R.-q., Zhao, D., Guo, C.-x., Zhu, A.-c., et al. (2020). Pathological mechanism of photodynamic therapy and photothermal therapy based on nanoparticles. *International journal of nanomedicine*, 6827–6838.

References

94. Austin, E., Wang, J. Y., Ozog, D. M., Zeitouni, N., Lim, H. W., & Jagdeo, J. (2025). Photodynamic therapy: overview and mechanism of action. *Journal of the American Academy of Dermatology*.
95. Correia, J. H., Rodrigues, J. A., Pimenta, S., Dong, T., & Yang, Z. (2021). Photodynamic therapy review: principles, photosensitizers, applications, and future directions. *Pharmaceutics, 13*(9), 1332.
96. Han, H., & Choi, K. (2021). Advances in Nanomaterial-Mediated Photothermal Cancer Therapies: Toward Clinical Applications. Biomedicines 2021, 9, 305. s Note: MDPI stays neutral with regard to jurisdictional claims in published ….
97. Fang, L., Chen, Z., Dai, J., Pan, Y., Tu, Y., Meng, Q., et al. (2025). Recent Advances in Strategies to Enhance Photodynamic and Photothermal Therapy Performance of Single-Component Organic Phototherapeutic Agents. *Advanced Science*, 2409157.
98. Duan, C., Yu, M., Xu, J., Li, B.-Y., Zhao, Y., & Kankala, R. K. (2023). Overcoming Cancer Multi-drug Resistance (MDR): Reasons, mechanisms, nanotherapeutic solutions, and challenges. *Biomedicine & Pharmacotherapy, 162*, 114643.
99. Chen, C., Wu, C., Yu, J., Zhu, X., Wu, Y., Liu, J., et al. (2022). Photodynamic-based combinatorial cancer therapy strategies: Tuning the properties of nanoplatform according to oncotherapy needs. *Coordination Chemistry Reviews, 461*, 214495.
100. Karmakar, A., Silswal, A., & Koner, A. L. (2024). Review of NIR-responsive "Smart"carriers for photothermal chemotherapy. *Journal of Materials Chemistry B, 12*(20), 4785–4808.
101. Carlos-Reyes, A., Muñiz-Lino, M. A., Romero-Garcia, S., López-Camarillo, C., & Hernández-de la Cruz, O. N. (2021). Biological adaptations of tumor cells to radiation therapy. *Frontiers in oncology, 11*, 718636.
102. Pan, S., Sun, Z., Zhao, B., Miao, L., Zhou, Q., Chen, T., et al. (2023). Therapeutic application of manganese-based nanosystems in cancer radiotherapy. *Biomaterials, 302*, 122321.
103. Ding, S., Chen, L., Liao, J., Huo, Q., Wang, Q., Tian, G., et al. (2023). Harnessing Hafnium-Based Nanomaterials for Cancer Diagnosis and Therapy. *Small, 19*(32), 2300341.
104. Zeng, H., Feng, H., Zhang, C., Kang, Z., Wu, J., Zhao, X., et al. (2025). Novel intravenous formulation for radiosensitization in osteosarcoma treatment. *Materials Today Bio, 32*, 101682.
105. Guo, R., Wang, S., Zhao, L., Zong, Q., Li, T., Ling, G., et al. (2022). Engineered nanomaterials for synergistic photo-immunotherapy. *Biomaterials, 282*, 121425.
106. Ji, B., Wei, M., & Yang, B. (2022). Recent advances in nanomedicines for photodynamic therapy (PDT)-driven cancer immunotherapy. *Theranostics, 12*(1), 434.
107. Xu, L., Liu, Y., Liu, F., Chen, Q., Li, M., Liao, N., et al. Tumor Cell-Derived Antigens for Cancer Immunotherapy. *Advanced Therapeutics*, e00113.
108. Zeng, Q., Ma, X., Song, Y., Chen, Q., Jiao, Q., & Zhou, L. (2022). Targeting regulated cell death in tumor nanomedicines. *Theranostics, 12*(2), 817.
109. Cai, Y., Chai, T., Nguyen, W., Liu, J., Xiao, E., Ran, X., et al. (2025). Phototherapy in cancer treatment: strategies and challenges. *Signal Transduction and Targeted Therapy, 10*(1), 115.

# Imaging, Diagnostics, and Theranostics Applications of Nanocrystals

## 6.1 Introduction

Cancer, a multifaceted group of diseases, is ranked globally as the second leading reason of mortality following cardiovascular disease, impacting a diverse range of individuals from children to adults [1, 2]. As per a report published by the WHO in 2020, cancer accounts for over 10 million deaths each year [3]. Continuous research is being carried out globally to develop novel tools and techniques to combat the current challenges and enhance the efficacy of cancer theranostics [3–6]. Recently, nanotechnology has gained significant attention, offering innovative strategies for detecting, diagnosing, preventing, and treating a wide range of diseases, including cancer [7, 8]. The application of nano-scaled particles, such as nanocrystals, polymeric, inorganic, lipid nanoparticles, liposomes, dendrimers, quantum dots, and carbon nanotubes, has revolutionized the field of medicine by enabling increasingly personalized diagnoses and treatments [9]. Among them, nanocrystals (NCs) have generated notable popularity due to their smaller size, larger surface area, and peculiar physicochemical properties, which allows them to target the tumor site, efficiently load drugs precisely, and control release, stimulation of drug solubility, and improved therapeutic potential while no noticeable negative effects on normal tissues [10–12].

Apart from targeted drug delivery, NCs have made significant advancements in cancer imaging modalities [13, 14]. Their peculiar magnetic and optical characteristics have revolutionized how we visualize and diagnose cancer, leading to high-resolution and sensitive imaging modalities [1]. Among the various forms of NCs, semiconductor quantum dots stand out due to their size-dependent fluorescence emission [15]. This characteristic allows them to emit light at specific wavelengths depending on their size, providing exceptional brightness and stability during imaging. As a result, quantum dots are excellent candidates for the precise visualization of tumors, improving the accuracy of cancer diagnosis [16]. Furthermore, by modifying the surfaces of these nanoparticles with targeting agents, they can be transformed into effective agents to enhance contrast in imaging tools. This modification helps ensure that the nanoparticles preferentially bind to cancer cells, enabling doctors to accurately diagnose, stage, and monitor the responses of tumors to treatment in real-time [1].

Integrating NCs with imaging techniques leads to innovative, multimodal cancer diagnosis and treatment approaches [17, 18]. This combination enhances the accuracy of cancer detection and allows for the development of personalized therapy strategies tailored to individual patient needs. NCs are a versatile platform incorporating various therapeutic agents within a single system. This capability enables the creation of synergistic effects, which can improve the effectiveness of the treatment by optimizing the drug ratios and ensuring targeted release at the site of interest [19]. As a result, this method enhances therapeutic efficacy while reducing systemic toxicity, a common side effect of traditional cancer treatments. Moreover, engineering NCs to react to external stimuli makes it possible to achieve controlled drug activation and spatiotemporal release [20, 21]. This feature allows the treatment to be fine-tuned, further personalizing the therapeutic approach based on the specific characteristics of the patient's cancer. The current chapter offers a complete overview of various applications of NCs for cancer theranostics. This analysis aims to highlight the practical effectiveness of NCs in real-life scenarios, demonstrating the potential of NCs to revolutionize cancer theranostics.

## 6.2 NCs in the Detection of Cancer Biomarkers

Detection of a tumor at an early stage for primary treatment has recently become an essential research topic, increasing the patient's survival rate [22]. Detection of cancer biomarkers, including proteins, carbohydrates, circulating tumor DNA, miRNA, etc. (Fig. 6.1) in blood or other body fluids allows early cancer detection and helps design therapy accordingly [23–25]. Recently, nanocrystals have emerged as pivotal tools in detecting cancer biomarkers, leveraging their unique properties to enhance sensitivity and specificity in diagnostic applications [26]. Various nanocrystals have been integrated into biosensing platforms, facilitating rapid and accurate identification of biomarkers associated with malignancies [27–29].

Qureshi et al. have developed a new point-of-care (PoC) diagnostic assay that utilizes multifunctional magnetic quantum dot (MQD) nanocrystals integrated into a bioactivated PoC chip designed to detect the hErbB2 biomarker protein in serum [30]. The MQDs consist of a central core made up of cadmium sulfide, cadmium selenide and zinc sulfide quantum dot nanocrystals, which are then coated with a thick layer of magnetic nanoparticles (MNPs).

When serum samples are applied to the PoC chip, the MQDs bind to the hErbB2 protein, creating a complex that can be easily isolated using a magnetic field. The assay

## 6.2 NCs in the Detection of Cancer Biomarkers

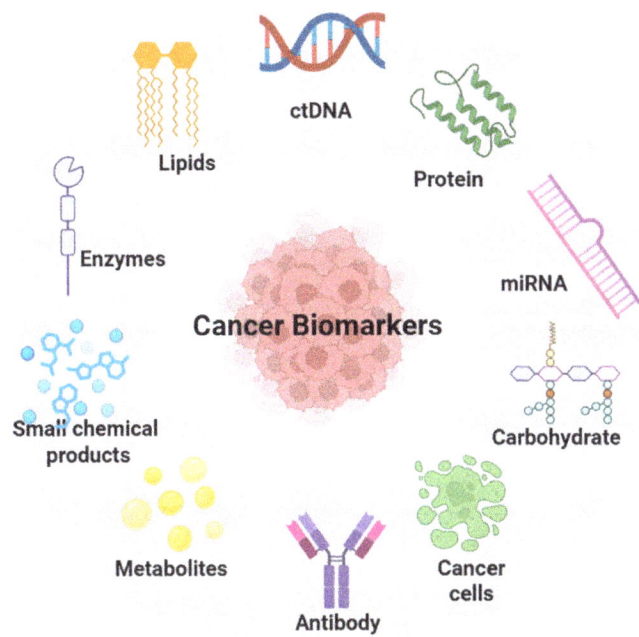

**Fig. 6.1** Scheme showing various cancer biomarkers. Created using BioRender

allows for direct visualization of the results. When illuminated with a hand-held UV torch, the complex fluoresces enable immediate detection within 30 min without needing complex equipment or additional reagents, allowing for results to be obtained rapidly and efficiently.

ctDNA (Circulating tumor DNA) is a vital cancer marker. Monitoring ctDNA plays a crucial role in the prognosis, detection, diagnosis, and treatment of cancer (Fig. 6.2) [31–33]. ctDNA are the DNA fragments released into the blood after the death or apoptosis of tumor cells [34, 35]. Therefore, for ultrasensitive detection of ctDNA Wang and team have developed a highly sensitive electrochemiluminescence (ECL) biosensor utilizing copper sulfide (CuS) colloidal nanocrystals (NCs) for the detection of ctDNA, a crucial biomarker in cancer management [34–36]. The detection range of the constructed ECL biosensor lies between 10 aM and 10 nM, and the detection limit (LOD) was found to be 2.74 aM.

The occurrence of protein-based biomarkers in the blood serum is widely explored for early recognition of disease and designing therapy accordingly. Carcinoembryonic antigen (CEA) is a serum protein that is identified as a main factor linked with different types of cancers, including breast, colon, lung, and ovarian [38–42]. Therefore, measuring serum CEA levels allows early diagnosis and effective treatment for cancer. Various techniques

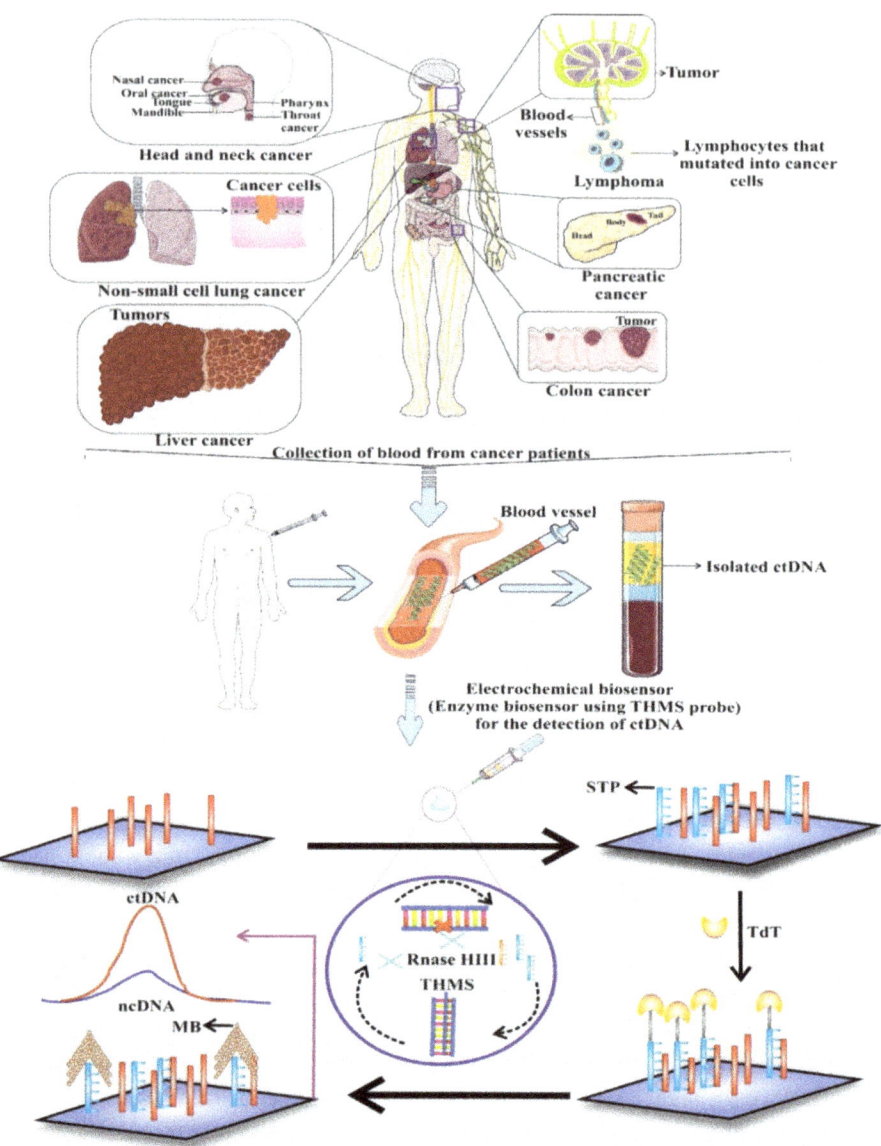

**Fig. 6.2** The figure shows the collection of blood samples from cancer patients, ct-DNA isolation, and identification of specific cancer through electrochemical biosensing [37]

have been employed to detect CEA level in blood serum, including optical trapping, radioimmunoassay, fluorescence and immunocytochemical method, nanobiosensor, field-effect transistor-based (FET-based), and plasmonic nanoimmunosensor [43]. However, these approaches have certain limitations, such as being time-consuming, posing radiation dangers, requiring complex procedures, and using expensive instruments. Hence, alternative strategies that are easy to utilize and have rapidity, portability, cost effectiveness accuracy are needed.

Currently, the identification of CEA via an electrochemical method has demonstrated great potential [44, 45]. However, a critical issue arises due to the reduced biocompatibility of the immobilization platform surface, resulting in reduced stability of the sensor. To overcome these challenges, Tran et al. have formed a novel three-dimensional system based on Cu-Au bimetallic NCs, which is integrated with carbon nanotubes that are grown over carbon spheres (Cu-Au/CNTs-CSs hybrid) for electrochemical sensing of CEA [43]. Cu-Au/CNTs-CSs hybrid can present numerous active sites and provides an outstanding system for immobilizing well-dispersed and highly dense anti-CEA to identify CEA sensitively. Cu-Au/CNTs-CSs hybrid demonstrated an improved electrochemical performance towards detection with higher sensitivity, a wide range of detection starting from 0.025 to 25 ng/mL, a lowest of detection at 0.5 pg/mL, and improved selectivity. The findings demonstrate that this sensor shows great potential to provide essential details for cancer diagnosis and management of cancer with excellent clinical outcomes.

MicroRNAs (miRNAs) expression patterns vary among normal and cancerous cells [46]. In each cancer type a specific type of miRNAs exist which gets overexpressed or downregulated in various body fluids [47]. These properties make detecting miRNAs a potential approach for early diagnosis, along with less invasive cancer monitoring [48].

Han and team have presented a photoluminescence-based strategy for the identification of miRNA biomarkers for multiple breast cancer using rare-earth-doped $CaF_2$ NCs. These NCs were mesoporous silica NPs whose surface was modified to retain photoluminescence, which allows DNA probe immobilization [49]. $CaF_2$ NCs were developed and modified with DNA probes, that has the ability to effectively detect biomarkers for breast cancer. This proposed approach can provide a quick, sensitive, simple, and selective detection of multiple miRNA, demonstrating potential for early cancer diagnosis applications.

## 6.3 NCs' Application in Imaging and Diagnosis of Cancer

It has been reported that nearly 7.6 million patients died of cancer in the last few years globally, and the number is expected to increase to 11.5 million by 2030, as per a report by the WHO [29]. Imaging plays a very crucial role in cancer diagnosis and therapy [50, 51]. It helps identify cancer size, stage, and tumor site, enabling doctors to design therapy accordingly. Although the field of medical science has shown tremendous improvement in recent decades, early-stage diagnosis and treatment for cancer remain challenging. In the majority of cases, cancer is detected when it has already reached the advanced stage, when conventional therapies such as chemotherapeutic drugs are less effective. In this context, the earlier detection via targeted and sustained imaging techniques for cancer diagnosis can significantly improve patient outcomes [29]. The imaging modalities currently utilized by medical practitioners for the early diagnosis and management of cancer include computed tomography (CT), single-photon emission computed tomography (SPECT), magnetic resonance imaging (MRI), optical imaging, x-ray plain film, PET, and ultrasound (US) [51, 52]. While these imaging techniques proved beneficial for imaging larger tumors, they fail to identify small clusters of cancer cells due to reduced sensitivity and resolution, which can lead to misdiagnosis and delayed treatment.

Essentially, while these imaging methods may work well for identifying larger tumors, they were not initially designed to detect small clusters of cancer cells, which can lead to missed diagnoses or delayed treatment. In the context of cancer, this limitation can hinder the effectiveness of screening programs and potentially impact patient outcomes [29, 53].

With the rapid advancement in molecular probes and nano field, imaging based diagnosis is deepening from conventional anatomical imaging to imaging at molecular level, that is real-time, highly specific, accurate, and and less-invasive, providing comprehensive information about cancerous cells [54–56]. Nanotechnology has significantly transformed cancer imaging techniques through NCs' applications because of their unique optical as well as magnetic properties, providing high-resolution and enhanced sensitivity [57]. High photo-stability along with size-dependent fluorescence emission is demonstrated by NCs in semiconductor quantum dots, making them outstanding candidates allowing precise visualization of tumor. In similar way, by modifications the NCs with targeting ligands, NCs can acts as contrast agents for improving the imaging modalities, allowing accurate diagnosis, identifying stage, and real-time observations of responses to the applied therapy [58, 59].

### 6.3.1 NCs in MRI

MRI is considered one among the most valuable, noninvasive, and effective bioimaging tools that provide high-resolution images [60]. Due to its reliability, superior spatial clarity, outstanding contrast in softer tissues, high signal-to-noise ratios, and absence of harmful rays. MRI creates three-dimensional images of particular organs and tissues using radio waves and a strong magnetic field [61–63]. Although MRI is popular diagnostic tools, due to its non-invasive and multidimensional tomographic properties combined with high spatial resolution, it has a limitation of low-signal sensitivity. Currently, nanocrystals, more specifically superparamagnetic nanocrystals, are widely explored for their role as an potential MR signal enhancer which can overcome the deawbacks of current MRI techniques [64].

## 6.3 NCs' Application in Imaging and Diagnosis of Cancer

Jia et al. have developed a metallic $Fe_2O_3$@CuFe-MOF NCs using copper and ferric metal that contains an organic framework, which is further embedded with ferric oxide. These NCs has the ability to act as contrast enhancer for effective in vivo diagnosis of prostate cancer using MRI [65]. 22RV1 tumor-bearing mice were injected with these synthesized NCs to assess its potential in diagnosis of prostate tumor. The $T_1$-weighted MR images of tumor sites collrected after 30 min of NCs exposure demonstrated brighter signal in the tumor site when compared to the untreated group.

Yang et al. developed oval-shaped, multi-crystalline manganese oxide (MCMO) nanocrystals of 200 nm diameter, as a novel MRI contrast agent to enhance the accuracy of tumor imaging [66]. An iRGD cyclopeptide was coupled to the MCMO (iRGD-pMCMO) surface to actively identify and accumulate in the tumor cells. After reaching the targeted site, the iRGD-pMCMO releases $Mn^{2+}$ ions due to and high-GSH (glutathione) and weakly acidic condition in the tumor microenvironment, allowing $Mn^{2+}$ ions to form interaction with cellular GSH, forming Mn-GSH chelates, allowing enhanced $T_1$-weighted MR contrast imaging (Fig. 6.3). Significantly enhanced $T_1$-weighted images in vivo demonstrated that iRGD-pMCMO can accurately diagnose both subcutaneous and orthotopic tumors. The T1 contrast effect of iRGD-pMCMO was found to be closely connected to the levels of GSH present in tumor cells.

The effects of iRGD-pMCMO as an MRI contrast were studied in vivo tumor models. When the tumor volume reached nearly 200 $mm^3$, the researchers injected pMCMO and iRGD-pMCMO into the tail vein of tumor-induced mice. It was observed that the $T_1$-weighted images of tumors brightened gradually with time in both the iRGD-pMCMO and pMCMO-treated mice (Fig. 6.4a). The brightest images for pMCMO and iRGD-pMCMO were seen at one and four hours post-injection, respectively, indicating both iRGD-pMCMO and pMCMO improved the tumor visibility in mice. However, the T1-weighted images of tumors in the group treated with iRGD-pMCMO were notably brighter when compared to the pMCMO group, highlighting more substantial tumor contrast effects of iRGD-pMCMO. The intensity of MRI signal of the tumors were examined employing microMRI software. Before injecting either of pMCMO or iRGD-pMCMO, the typical MRI signal intensity of the tumors was approximately 140 units. However, after two hours, the signal intensity reached 185 units in the pMCMO group, whereas an increased signal intensity of 229 units was observed in the iRGD-pMCMO group after 4 h (Fig. 6.4b). This indicates iRGD-pMCMO enhances the contrast more effectively and maintains a higher tumor signal over time compared to pMCMO, making it a promising contrast agent for improved MRI in clinical settings.

### 6.3.2 NCs in CT

Computed tomography (CT) is another popular diagnostic imaging technique that utilizes X-rays to develop a 3-dimensional depiction of the anatomy in living animals [67]. CT can

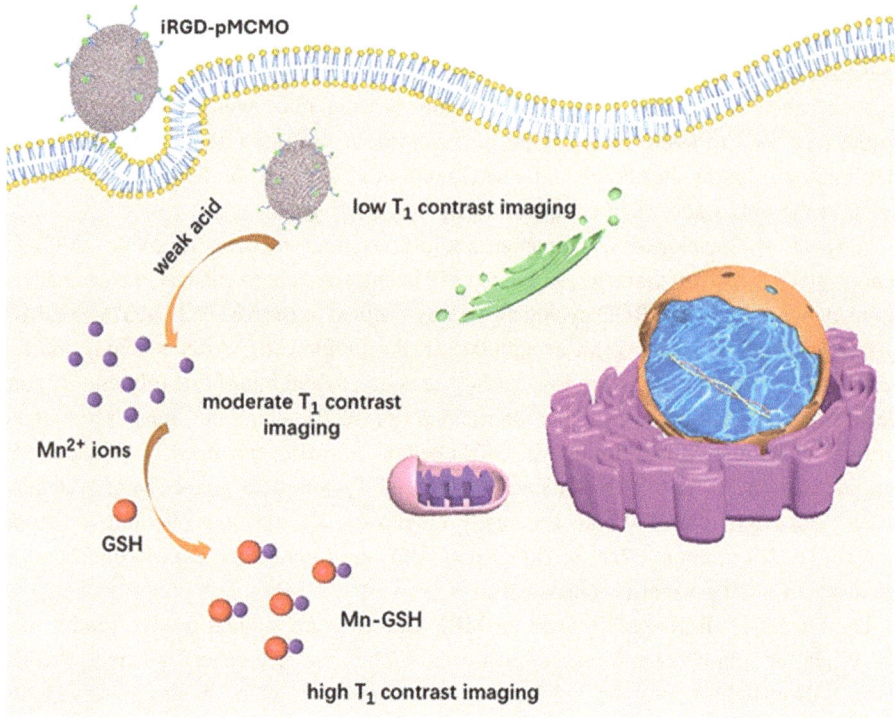

**Fig. 6.3** Graphical representation of the role of iRGD-pMCMO as a contrast agent in MRI [66]

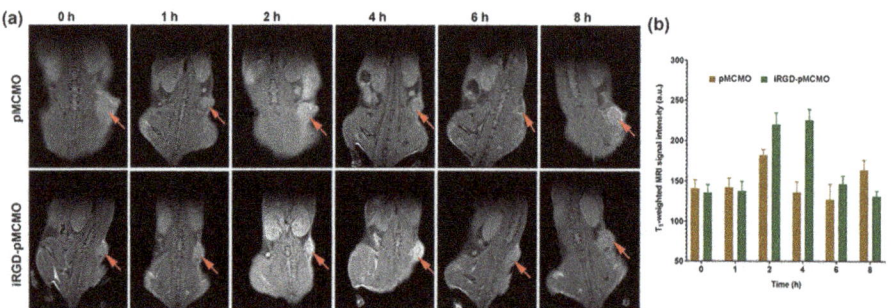

**Fig. 6.4** The research displays **a** T1-weighted MRI scans and **b** the associated tumor signal intensity in PC-3 tumor-bearing mice at the coronal section after administering pMCMO and iRGD-pMCMO treatments. The tumor site is marked by red arrows in the images. *$p < 0.05$ [66]

## 6.3 NCs' Application in Imaging and Diagnosis of Cancer

be employed in any stage of the diagnostic process, starting from detection, to differentiation, to evaluation of tumor extension and staging [68]. CT is an efficient, non-invasive clinical in vivo imaging strategy for obtaining real-time images of internal organs. It is widely used for the screening of lung, colon, neck, head, breast cancers, etc. with an accurate spatial and temporal tumor imaging, enabling in follow-up biopsy procedures, surgeries, radio- radio-chemo-therapies, etc [69]. Unfortunately, due to the lack of natural contrast between different tissues, CT imaging often requires contrast agents to improve the visibility of a specific site in the body under X-ray.

Wu et al. have developed lanthanide-based nanocrystals for lymph node CT imaging [68]. They injected 150 µL of NCs (4.0 mg mL$^{-1}$) into the left paw of the mice for lymph node imaging. CT images captured post 20 min of injection demonstrated a notable contrast improvement of the lymph node, indicating a potential role of lanthanide-based nanocrystals in X-ray CT imaging.

Jia and team have designed a biocompatible albumin-directed platinum (Pt@BSA) NCs of 2.1 mm core size for exploring its utility in CT imaging [70]. They compared the X-ray attenuation ability of Pt@BSA to Ultravist, a popular contrast. The in vitro CT scans of Ultravist and the Pt@BSA demonstrated brighter CT images in both groups. However, the contrast effect of Pt@BSA was found to be more reinforced than Ultravist, showing nearly 2.4-fold higher Hounsfield units (HUs) than Ultravist at a similar concentration of 12 mM. The potential of Pt@BSA nanocrystals as contrast agents was further investigated for in vivo CT imaging. A volume of 200 µL containing Pt at a concentration of 10 mg mL$^{-1}$ was intravenously administered into a tumor-bearing mouse model through the tail vein. CT images were acquired at various time points, ranging from 5 min to 24 h post-injection. For comparison, mice injected with Ultravist were included in the study. The steady increase in uptake of the Pt@BSA in key organs was observed. The reconstructed 3D (Fig. 6.5a and b) and 2D coronal (Fig. 6.5c and d) images show this accumulation highlighted in different colors. The difference in corresponding CT values of the heart, liver, kidney, and bladder was quantitatively analyzed over time after the administration of Pt@BSA. The contrast values of the heart and liver were found to be enhanced in the Pt@BSA group just after 5 min of injection. In contrast, no such enhancement was observed in the Ultravist group (Fig. 6.6). The CT value for the liver was found to increase with time, showing a peak of $111 \pm 6$ HU after 1 h of injection, before gradually dropping back to its prior level ($76 \pm 4$ HU) indicating Pt@BSA nanocrystals are taken up by macrophages in the liver, that can be useful for diagnosing liver-related diseases. The contrast of heart reached a peak of $58 \pm 2$ HU at 5 min, after which it slowly declined over 4 h and then returned to a normal level of $44 \pm 3$ HU, suggesting that Pt@BSA nanocrystals might enhance the visualization of blood vessels for a more extended period of time that is valuable for angiography. All the above findings demonstrate that Pt@BSA nanocrystals significantly improve the contrast in CT scans, making them a promising tool for imaging applications of tumor tissues in vivo.

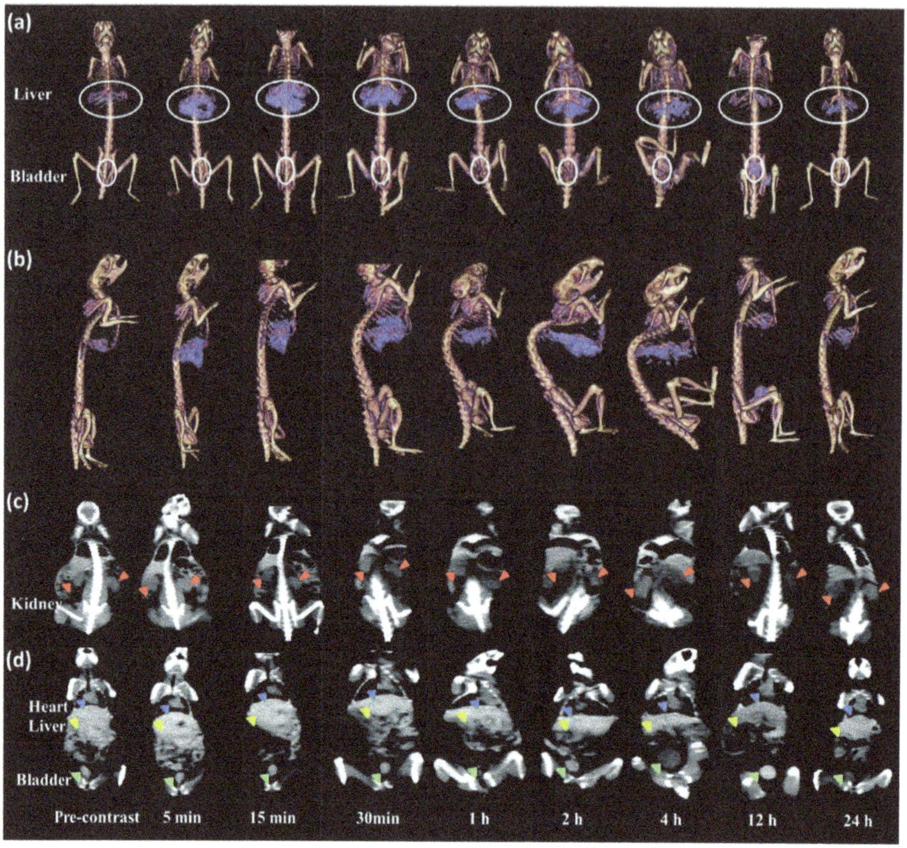

**Fig. 6.5** CT scans showing a mouse (**a** and **b**) and coronal views highlighting the kidney (**c**), heart, liver, and bladder (**d**) taken before and after the intravenous injection of Pt@BSA NCs at various time points. (red, blue, yellow, and green denote kidney, heart, liver, and bladder, respectively) [70]

**Fig. 6.6** HU of various tissues before and after administration of Pt@BSA NCs at different time point (*$P < 0.05$) [70]

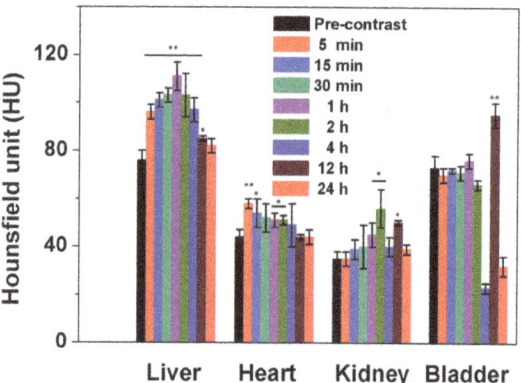

## 6.3.3 NCs in Fluorescent Imaging

Since last few decades, fluorescence imaging has developed significant interest as a complementary medical technique for cancer diagnosis, enabling the detection of tumor tissues with a high spatio-temporal resolution in clinical studies [71]. Currently, NIR (near-infrared) fluorophores are gaining popularity in medical imaging, providing wide-field and real-time imaging abilities, enabling high-resolution bioimaging [72, 73]. Unfortunately, the fluorophores have certain limitations, including limited solubility in an aqueous environment, short lifetimes in vivo circulation, and low quantum efficiencies. To overcome these drawbacks, researchers are exploring innovative approaches such as encapsulating the fluorophore inside a nanoparticle or attaching it to the surface of the nanoparticle [74]. Nanoparticle-based NIR fluorophores can address many drawbacks associated with traditional NIR organic dyes, including issues like low solubility in water, insufficient quantum yield, limited sensitivity for detection, poor photostability, reduced stability within biological environments, and weak capabilities for multiplexing [75].

Zhang and team have successfully developed the c(RGDfC) coupled erbium-based NCs (ErNPs@cRGD), demonstrating optical properties in the NIR-II region (1500–1700 nm) [72]. They intravenously administered ErNPs, both functionalized and non-functionalized with the c(RGDfC) peptide, to BALB/c mice with subcutaneous tumors to investigate the in vivo tumor-targeting effectiveness of ErNPs@cRGD. The results of NIR-II bioimaging showed a gradual increase in SBRs over time, peaking at 24 h after administration in the ErNPs@cRGD mice. Whereas, the group treated with ErNPs modified with poly (ethylene glycol) (ErNPs@PEG) only demonstrated an increase in SBRs up to 12 h post-injection (Fig. 6.7a and b). This indicates ErNPs@cRGD allowed for deeper tissue penetration and more effective targeting of tumors. As a result, the NIR-II fluorescence imaging using ErNPs@cRGD provided improved visualization of tumors, enhancing the thoroughness of tumor removals, detecting several microtumors, and differentiating malignant tissues from healthy ones in different mouse models.

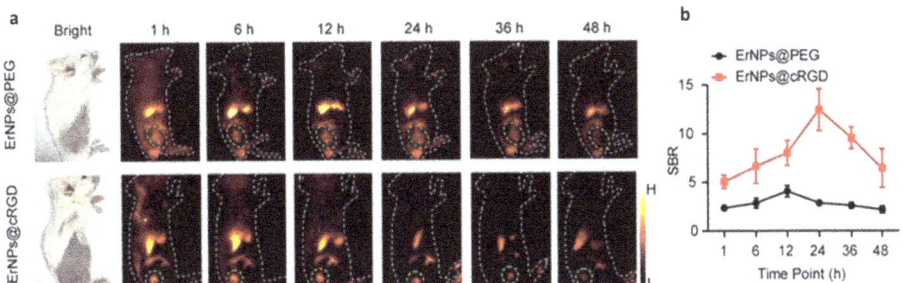

**Fig. 6.7** **a** Bright-field and NIR-IIb fluorescence images and **b** the signal-to-background ratios (SBRs) of mice treated with ErNPs@PEG and ErNPs@cRGD [72]

Another group, Hu et al., have developed a novel carrier system using polydopamine and cellulose nanocrystals (PDA@CNC) for targeted fluorescence imaging of tumor cells. Inhibitors of microRNA-21 (miRNAi) were successfully integrated into PDA@CNC to create a multifunctional nanocomposite known as FAM-miRNAi@PDA@CNC. This NCs was designed to aid in situ fluorescence imaging of tumor biomarkers in breast cancer cells. The elevated levels of miRNA-21 in breast cancer cells interact with the FAM-miRNAi, triggering green fluorescence of FAM to recognize breast cancer cells [76]. The researchers studied the effects of the incubation period on miRNA-21 imaging. They found enhanced FAM fluorescence in cells after incubating NCs with MCF-7 cells for 3 h, suggesting successful binding of the NCs to the cancer cells.

### 6.3.4 NCs in Multimodal Imaging of Cancer

Multimodal bioimaging integrates the advantages of utilizing multiple imaging methods, including various types of microscopy (such as electron, light, and atomic force), molecular imaging techniques (like fluorescence, PET, and bioluminescence), structural imaging approaches (including X-ray CT, MRI, and ultrasound), and spectroscopy (such as magnetic resonance, infrared, and Raman). By combining different modalities, researchers can address the limitations of a single technique, leading to a more comprehensive understanding of the sample being studied [77].

Fan et al. have designed a lanthanide-based nanocrystal doped with $^{177}Lu^{3+}$ that shows both time-resolved optical imaging and SPECT (Single Photon Emission Computed Tomography) imaging abilities to facilitate long-term, non-invasive in vivo trafficking of nanomaterials metabolism [78]. Both optical imaging and SPECT are advanced techniques used to visualize the distribution of nanoparticles inside a living system. SPECT gives a high-resolution, 3D visualization allowing detailed assessment of nanoparticle distribution across various organs over time. Optical imaging provides highly sensitive 2D images. Optical imaging techniques can detect even minor pulmonary accumulation of nanoparticles, which is not detectable by SPECT/CT, indicating higher sensitivity of optical imaging for identifying even weak luminescent signals. Meanwhile, SPECT generates excellent 3D anatomical images, unaffected by depth-dependent attenuation or tissue scattering, providing a comprehensive evaluation of nanoparticle biodistribution.

Jiang et al. have studied the potential of $CuFeSe_2$ NCs for multimodal imaging [79]. Researchers intravenously administered $CuFeSe_2$ NCs into 4T1 tumor-bearing mice to examine whether the deposition $CuFeSe_2$ NCs via the EPR (enhanced permeability and retention) effect would be sufficient for the multimodal imaging of tumors in vivo. First, PA (photoacoustic) images captured at different time points after injection demonstrated that the brightness of the tumor site enhanced significantly, reaching its peak around 4 h postinjection. The peak tumor signal was almost double that of the control level, indicating that there was a buildup of NCs in the tumor. Additionally, the same dosage of

CuFeSe$_2$ NCs was administered intravenously to mice with 4T1 tumors, and CT images were recorded at various time intervals. Unlike the findings of PAI, the CT images demonstrated no enhancement, indicating minimum accumulation of NCs in the tumors. However, the study highlighted the excellent imaging capability of NCs when administered intratumorally compared to a commercial contrast agent, iopromide. In this case, both agents were administered into the same mouse at an equal 25 mg/kg dose at two separate tumor sites. The results demonstrated a marked improvement in imaging performance for CuFeSe$_2$ NCs, which yielded a CT value of 349.23 HU, compared to only 65.69 HU for iopromide. The above findings indicate that CuFeSe$_2$ NCs are up-and-coming candidates for multimodal imaging applications, particularly when sufficient accumulation in the target lesion can be achieved.

## 6.4 NCs in the Cancer Theranostics

Cancer theranostics is a broad term that combines both diagnosis and therapy for cancer, allowing early diagnosis, accurate molecular imaging, targeted therapy, precise treatment at the correct dose and time, followed by real-time monitoring of treatment efficacy [80, 81]. It accelerates the development of novel drugs with minimum side effects, improved disease management, and reduced cost. Cancer patients are in great need of such investigation for rapid diagnosis and treatment [82].

Cauda and team have designed an acoustically driven hybrid NC to treat pancreatic ductal adenocarcinoma (PDAC) [83]. PDAC exhibits inherent resistance to chemotherapy, a non-immunogenic tumor microenvironment, a dense fibrous stroma, and low oxygen levels, all of which impede drug delivery to the tumor [84, 85]. Cauda's team has proposed a multimodal approach that utilizes nanoparticles (NPs) of zinc oxide (ZnO) that are iron-doped and coated with lipids, activated by an ultrasound transducer. While ZnO NPs were used for their anti-cancerous abilities, iron was added as a doping agent that ensures ZnO remains intrinsically safe unless activated by ultrasound [86–88]. The group studied the synergistic effect of iron-doped ZnO NPs, enhancing a fluorescent sonosensitizer combined with local ultrasound stimulation for the treatment of PDAC. The formed NPs were combined with AlexaFluor, which allows for real-time tracking of their localization in vivo, followed by intratumoral administration to a murine model for PDAC to improve bioavailability at the tumor site and reduce off-target effects of systemic delivery. The sonosensitizer-enhanced NCs, in combination with ultrasound, significantly increased ROS generation that reduced the viability of KPC cells. The results demonstrated a dual cytotoxic action, causing shrinkage and apoptosis of the tumor due to the recruitment of immune cells to the tumor site. Additionally, the mice exposed to these hybrid NCs in coupled with ultrasound demonstrated prolonged survival when compared to the control, highlighting the theranostic potential of hybrid NCs (Fig. 6.8).

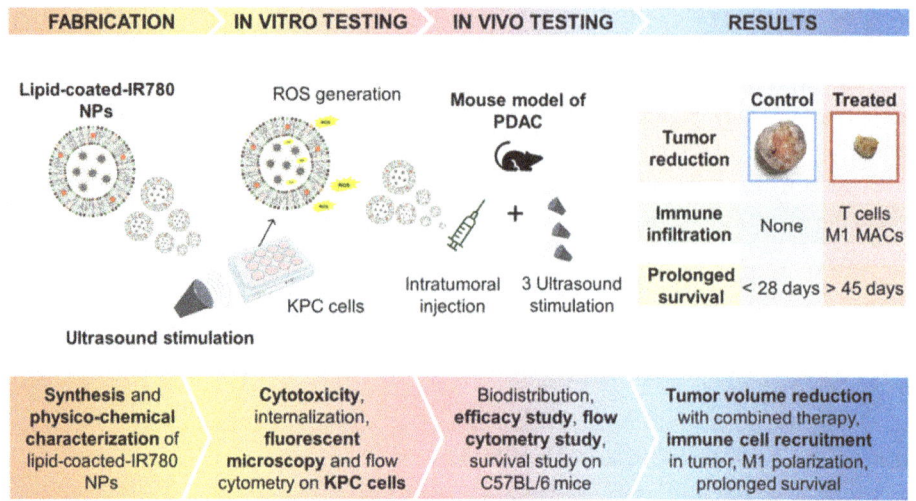

**Fig. 6.8** Scheme showing the effects of PDAC NCs under US in treating cancer [83]

Moon and co-workers have developed a multifunctional mesoporous silica nanoparticle (MSN) for combination immunotherapy [89]. The synthesized MSNs were simultaneously loaded with CpG oligodeoxynucleotide (CpG ODN), a strong agonist of Toll-like receptor-9, and the photosensitizer chlorin e6 (Ce6) for a combined photodynamic therapy and immunotherapy approach. Furthermore, the surface of the MSNs was modified with a neoantigen peptide designed to be rapidly cleaved within the intracellular environment of tumors. The results of PET and radioisotope $^{64}$Cu demonstrated that neoantigens conjugated to MSNs were effectively accumulated in the tumor site post intravenous (i.v.) administration. When PDT was subsequently applied, it promoted the recruitment of dendritic cells to the tumor areas, causing activation of strong neoantigen-specific CD8α + cytotoxic T lymphocyte responses. In examining the impact of individual treatments like PDT or vaccination on their own, it was found that the combination of PDT and personalized cancer vaccination produced a significant synergy. This combination not only demonstrated potent antitumor efficacy against localized tumors but also had significant effects on distant tumors across multiple murine tumor models, highlighting the promising potential of this combined approach for the treating advanced cancer.

Liver cancer is another common global malignancy with more than 0.9 million cases annually as per Global Cancer Statistics 2020 [90]. Hepatocellular carcinoma (HCC) is often identified at a later stage, resulting in a high mortality rate, demanding novel and effective diagnosis and treatment strategies [91, 92]. Therefore, Xing et al. have developed a novel multifunctional nanomaterial, UMFNPs/Ce6@MBs, that is coupled with chlorin e6 (Ce6) and ultra-small manganese ferrite NPs (UMFNPs) [93]. The

UMFNPs/Ce6@MBs were further integrated into a combination of sonodynamic therapy and photodynamic therapy (SPDT) for the treatment of hepatocellular carcinoma (HCC) (Scheme 6.1). These nanoparticles display biodegradability that is sensitive to both $H_2O_2$ and pH levels, enabling the release of UMFNPs and the photosensitizer Ce6 within the tumor microenvironment (TME), while also producing $O_2$ and $Mn^{2+}$. The released $Mn^{2+}$ ion nanoparticles can serve as T1 contrast agents for MRI of mice with tumors, while the released Ce6 provides improved fluorescence imaging features. Researchers found that UMFNPs/Ce6@MBs exhibit a synergistic effect between sonodynamic therapy and photodynamic therapy, facilitated by multi-modal near-infrared fluorescence imaging and contrast-enhanced ultrasound (CEUS) monitoring. This highlights their significant potential for precise diagnosis and treatment assistance in liver cancer.

As per the findings of the WHO, the fifth most common form of cancer reported globally is the skin carcinoma [94, 95]. In 2022, the American Academy of Dermatology (AAD) 2022 disclosed that nearly every day in the United States, 9,500 individuals receive a diagnosis of skin cancer [96]. For the treatment of skin cancer, Borlan et al. have developed a dual-modal organic-nanoagent for enhancing photothermal therapy (PTT) and Sentinel Lymph Node Biopsy (SLNB) procedures in patients [97]. PTT is a well-known cancer therapeutic strategy that uses heat to eradicate tumorous cells [98–100]. SLNB procedures is utilized to determine if cancer has spread from its initial location [101, 102]. In

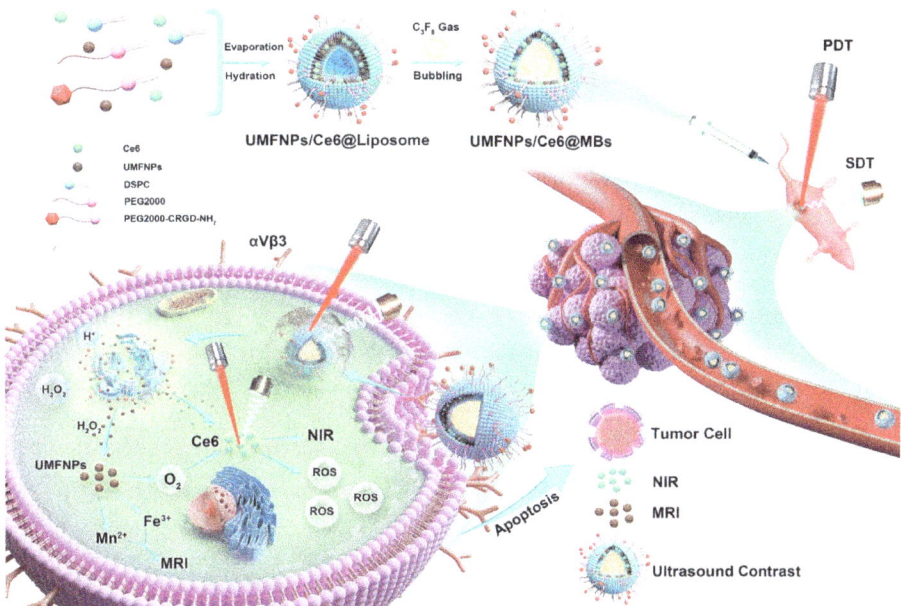

**Scheme 6.1** Illustrative diagram showing the process for creating UMFNPs/Ce6@MBs and the way they function in the treatment of HCC [93]

their work, Borlan et al. encapsulated NIR-797-isothiocyanate inside a poly(D, L-lactide-co-glycolide) acid (PLGA) NCs of 270 nm diameter with 60% NIR-797 loading ability. The nanoreagent showed excellent fluorescence properties along with efficient light-to-heat conversion, which is essential for PTT. The in vivo effectiveness of the formemed NCs as photothermal agents was studied in a murine model. 4 h post administration of NCs, the model was exposed to 808 nm medical laser for 8 min, and the temperature change was monitored. Mild hyperthermia with 43.8 °C temperatures was observed at the tumor site. Ex vivo microscopy of tissue samples collected from tumor sites demonstrated the persistence of fluorescent signal from NIR-797–loaded PLGA NCs, and they were found to be uniformly distributed in the tissue samples. Further, Imaging-guided photodynamic therapy (IgPDT) has gained notable interest as a promising theragnostic approach that combines both diagnosis and treatment of cancer. It allows cancer treatment while simultaneously providing real-time diagnostic bioimage [104–106]. In contrast to the traditional PDT, IgPDT provides more precise controllability, real-time diagnosis, increased therapeutic accuracy, and negligible side effects. Additionally, it shows its photoactivity only after being taken up by the cancer cells, protecting the healthy cells [107–109]. Kim et al. have developed LaB-Br NPs that are capable of destroying hepatocellular carcinoma cells when exposed to red light, while also allowing for fluorescence cell imaging during this phototherapeutic period [110]. The dual fluorescence photosensitizing property of the synthesized LaB-Br NPs can be switched off. Particularly at the time of NPs synthesis, the fluorescence and singlet oxygen generation are temporarily paused. However, after getting inside, the paused activities resume, causing apoptosis of cancer cells.

Another group of researchers, Xiao and team, have developed cationic antineoplastic anticancer nanoparticles (mt-NP$^{Bodipy}$).[103] These NPs are designed to specifically target and destroy the cell membranes of cancer cells after NIR light exposure for NIR-II fluorescence bio-imaging, PDT, and photo-immunotherapy. Moreover, mt-NP$^{Bodipy}$ can produce a large amount of ROS upon light exposure for a longer time, causing lipid peroxidation, inducing membrane destabilization, resulting in photodynamic immunotherapy. In vivo experiments showed that mt-NPBodipy produced strong NIR-II fluorescence signals, which are essential for NIR-II bioimaging. It was also observed that the combination of mt-NPBodipy and L effectively inhibited the growth of CT26 tumors without causing significant side effects. Furthermore, this combination enhances the recruitment of dendritic cells (DCs) and elevates the levels of antigen-specific cytotoxic T lymphocytes (CTLs) within the tumor microenvironment (TME), leading to a reprogramming of the immunosuppressive TME and promoting antitumor immune responses (Fig. 6.9).

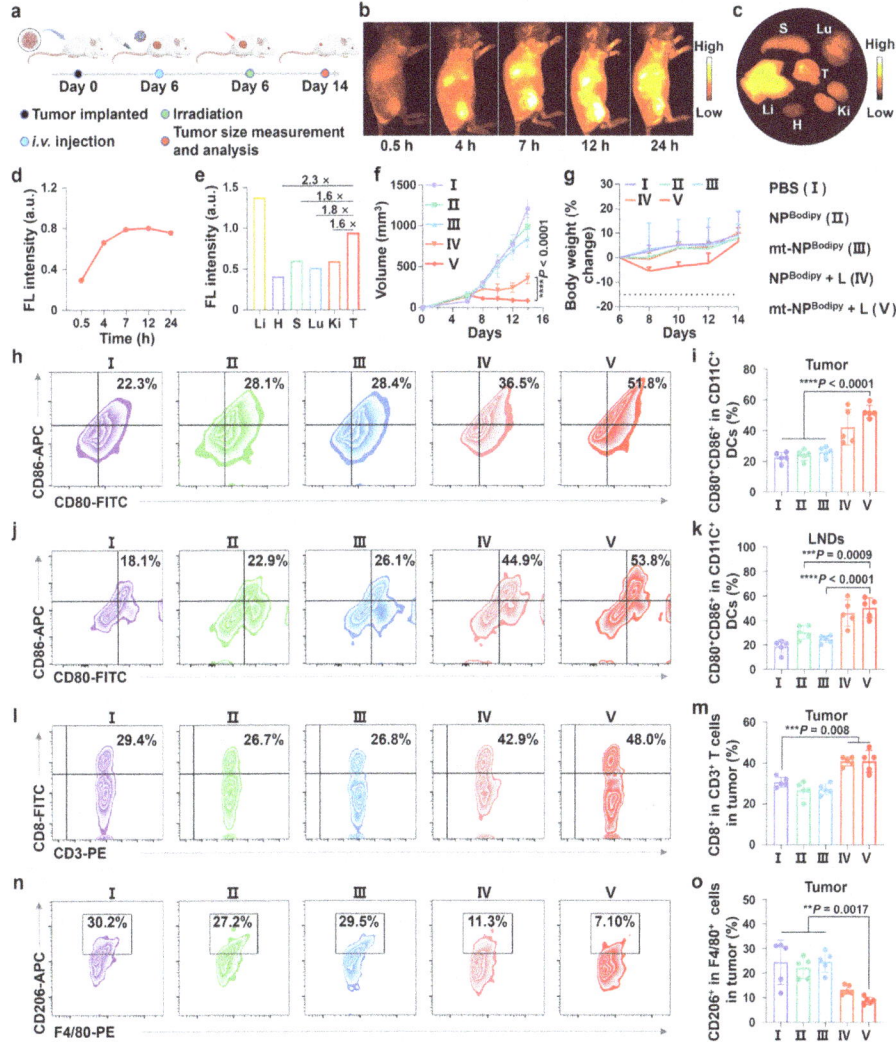

**Fig. 6.9 a** A diagram depicting a CT26 tumor-bearing mouse model that was treated with mt-NPBodipy + L. NIR-II fluorescence bioimaging was performed on **b** mice receiving mt-NPBodipy at various time intervals, and **c** the main tissues and organs (T for tumor, Lu for lung, H for heart, S for spleen, L for liver, Ki for kidney) were collected after 24 h by euthanizing the mice. A semi-quantitative assessment of NIR-II fluorescence **d** in the tumor regions at different time points and **e** in the organs after 24 h was conducted. Additionally, **f** tumor growth inhibition curves were generated, along with **g** a graph showing weight changes. Flow cytometry analysis included **h** FCM plot and **i** the quantification of dendritic cells identified as CD11c$^+$ within the tumor tissues. **j** Another FCM plot illustrated **k** the quantification of CD80$^+$ CD86$^+$ dendritic cells gated on CD11c$^+$ cells within the lymph nodes. **l** An additional FCM plot led to **m** the quantification of CD$^{8+}$ T cells gated on CD$^{3+}$ cells in the tumorous tissues. Lastly, **n** another FCM plot provided **o** the quantification of M2 macrophages (identified as CD206 + gated on F4/80 + cells) within the tumor tissues. *$p < 0.05$ [103]

## 6.5 Conclusion

NCs have achieved significant popularity in the domain of cancer theranostics, providing greater advantages than the traditional approaches for cancer diagnosis and treatment. Nanosized nanocarriers (NCs) facilitate the precise, targeted delivery of therapeutic agents to tumor sites, enabling the controlled release of these agents. This advanced delivery system also mitigates potential side effects on adjacent cells and tissues, enhancing the overall efficacy and safety of cancer treatments. The distinctive optical properties of nanoparticles (NCs) have brought about a paradigm shift in cancer tissue imaging, enhancing sensitivity and producing high-resolution images. This advancement enables effective staging, accuracy in diagnosis, and real-time observation of responses to the treatment approach. The conjugation of NCs with different imaging methods opens the way for multimodal strategies, enabling comprehensive detection, diagnosis, and development of personalized cancer therapy.

## References

1. Patel, A., Patel, K., Patel, V., Rajput, M. S., Patel, R., & Rajput, A. (2024). Nanocrystals: an emerging paradigm for cancer therapeutics. *Future Journal of Pharmaceutical Sciences, 10*(1), 4, https://doi.org/10.1186/s43094-024-00579-4.
2. Mani, K., Deng, D., Lin, C., Wang, M., Hsu, M. L., & Zaorsky, N. G. (2024). Causes of death among people living with metastatic cancer. *Nature Communications, 15*(1), 1519, https://doi.org/10.1038/s41467-024-45307-x.
3. Beg, S., & Rahman, M. (2022). Nanomedicine for Cancer: Targeted Therapy, Vaccination, Pharmacokinetics, and Challenges. *Current Drug Metabolism, 23*(8), 586–586.
4. Mandan, J., & Kanugo, A. (2025). Recent Advancements in Nanoparticles-based Approaches for the Theranostics of Glioblastoma Multiforme. *Current Pharmaceutical Biotechnology*.
5. Singh, S., Gupta, A., & Varshney, M. (2025). Application of Nanotechnology as a Novel Approach to the Treatment of Skin Cancer. *Current Bioactive Compounds, 21*(3), E200524230100.
6. Naik, G. A. R. R., Rachana, S., Colaco, V., Hedayat, P., Roy, A. A., Pokale, R., et al. (2025). Silica and Non-Silica-Based Core-Shell Nanoconstructs for Cancer Theragnostics. In *Core-Shell Nano Constructs for Cancer Theragnostic: Current Scenario, Challenges and Regulatory Aspects* (pp. 453–493): Springer.
7. Theivendren, P., Kunjiappan, S., Pavadai, P., Ravi, K., Murugavel, A., Dayalan, A., et al. (2025). Revolutionizing Cancer Immunotherapy: Emerging Nanotechnology-Driven Drug Delivery Systems for Enhanced Therapeutic Efficacy. *ACS Measurement Science Au, 5*(1), 31–55, https://doi.org/10.1021/acsmeasuresciau.4c00062.
8. Wang, B., Hu, S., Teng, Y., Chen, J., Wang, H., Xu, Y., et al. (2024). Current advance of nanotechnology in diagnosis and treatment for malignant tumors. *Signal Transduction and Targeted Therapy, 9*(1), 200, https://doi.org/10.1038/s41392-024-01889-y.

9. Chura, S. S. D., Sudo, K. A., Quintão Arantes Faria, J. A., Borges, G. S. M., & Carneiro, G. (2024). 2 - Nanoencapsulation approaches for enhancing cancer therapy. In S. Nimesh, N. Gupta, & G. Carneiro (Eds.), *Cancer Therapy* (pp. 13–42): Elsevier.
10. Miao, X., Yang, W., Feng, T., Lin, J., & Huang, P. (2018). Drug nanocrystals for cancer therapy. *WIREs Nanomedicine and Nanobiotechnology, 10*(3), e1499, https://doi.org/10.1002/wnan.1499.
11. Navya, P. N., Kaphle, A., Srinivas, S. P., Bhargava, S. K., Rotello, V. M., & Daima, H. K. (2019). Current trends and challenges in cancer management and therapy using designer nanomaterials. *Nano Convergence, 6*(1), 23, https://doi.org/10.1186/s40580-019-0193-2.
12. Zhao, J., Du, J., Wang, J., An, N., Zhou, K., Hu, X., et al. (2021). Folic Acid and Poly(ethylene glycol) Decorated Paclitaxel Nanocrystals Exhibit Enhanced Stability and Breast Cancer-Targeting Capability. *ACS Appl Mater Interfaces, 13*(12), 14577–14586, https://doi.org/10.1021/acsami.1c00184.
13. Chen, W., Huang, J., Guo, Y., Wang, X., Lin, Z., Wei, R., et al. (2025). Nanocrystals for Intravenous Drug Delivery: Composition Development, Preparation Methods and Applications in Oncology. *AAPS PharmSciTech, 26*(3), 66, https://doi.org/10.1208/s12249-025-03064-0.
14. Du, S., Wu, K., Guan, Y., Lin, X., Gao, S., Huang, S., et al. (2025). Biomimetic celastrol nanocrystals with enhanced efficacy and reduced toxicity for suppressing breast cancer invasion and metastasis. *Int J Pharm, 671*, 125221, https://doi.org/10.1016/j.ijpharm.2025.125221.
15. Park, H., Shin, D. J., & Yu, J. (2021). Categorization of Quantum Dots, Clusters, Nanoclusters, and Nanodots. *Journal of Chemical Education, 98*(3), 703–709, https://doi.org/10.1021/acs.jchemed.0c01403.
16. Fang, M., Peng, C. W., Pang, D. W., & Li, Y. (2012). Quantum dots for cancer research: current status, remaining issues, and future perspectives. *Cancer Biol Med, 9*(3), 151–163, https://doi.org/10.7497/j.issn.2095-3941.2012.03.001.
17. Rashidi, N., Davidson, M., Apostolopoulos, V., & Nurgali, K. (2024). Nanoparticles in cancer diagnosis and treatment: Progress, challenges, and opportunities. *Journal of Drug Delivery Science and Technology, 95*, 105599, https://doi.org/10.1016/j.jddst.2024.105599.
18. Wang, T., Ni, Y., & Liu, L. (2024). Innovative Imaging Techniques for Advancing Cancer Diagnosis and Treatment. *Cancers (Basel), 16*(14), https://doi.org/10.3390/cancers16142607.
19. Joseph, E., & Singhvi, G. (2019). Chapter 4 - Multifunctional nanocrystals for cancer therapy: a potential nanocarrier. In A. M. Grumezescu (Ed.), *Nanomaterials for Drug Delivery and Therapy* (pp. 91–116): William Andrew Publishing.
20. Qiao, Y., Wan, J., Zhou, L., Ma, W., Yang, Y., Luo, W., et al. (2019). Stimuli-responsive nanotherapeutics for precision drug delivery and cancer therapy. *Wiley Interdiscip Rev Nanomed Nanobiotechnol, 11*(1), e1527, https://doi.org/10.1002/wnan.1527.
21. Mura, S., Nicolas, J., & Couvreur, P. (2013). Stimuli-responsive nanocarriers for drug delivery. *Nature Materials, 12*(11), 991–1003, https://doi.org/10.1038/nmat3776.
22. Sravanthi Peddinti, A., Maloji, S., & Manepalli, K. (2021). Evolution in diagnosis and detection of brain tumor – review. *Journal of Physics: Conference Series, 2115*(1), 012039, https://doi.org/10.1088/1742-6596/2115/1/012039.
23. Pessoa, L. S., Heringer, M., & Ferrer, V. P. (2020). ctDNA as a cancer biomarker: A broad overview. *Crit Rev Oncol Hematol, 155*, 103109, https://doi.org/10.1016/j.critrevonc.2020.103109.
24. Zhang, Y., Li, M., Gao, X., Chen, Y., & Liu, T. (2019). Nanotechnology in cancer diagnosis: progress, challenges and opportunities. *Journal of Hematology & Oncology, 12*(1), 137, https://doi.org/10.1186/s13045-019-0833-3.

25. Tenchov, R., Sapra, A. K., Sasso, J., Ralhan, K., Tummala, A., Azoulay, N., et al. (2024). Biomarkers for Early Cancer Detection: A Landscape View of Recent Advancements, Spotlighting Pancreatic and Liver Cancers. *ACS Pharmacology & Translational Science, 7*(3), 586–613, https://doi.org/10.1021/acsptsci.3c00346.
26. Shahazi, R., Saddam, A. I., Islam, M. R., Rahman, M. M., Paimard, G., Kumer, A., et al. (2024). Recent progress in Nanomaterial based biosensors for the detection of cancer biomarkers in human fluids. *Nano Carbons, 2*(2), 1254–1254.
27. Yang, Y., Zeng, J., Shu, Y., & Gao, Q. (2020). Revealing facet effects of palladium nanocrystals on electrochemical biosensing. *ACS Appl Mater Interfaces, 12*(13), 15622–15630.
28. Song, J., Huang, P., Duan, H., & Chen, X. (2015). Plasmonic vesicles of amphiphilic nanocrystals: optically active multifunctional platform for cancer diagnosis and therapy. *Accounts of chemical research, 48*(9), 2506–2515.
29. Misra, K. P., & Misra, R. (2023). ZnO-based quantum dots for biosensing, cancer imaging and Therapy: an overview. *Biomedical Materials & Devices, 1*(1), 99–107.
30. Qureshi, A., Tufani, A., Corapcioglu, G., & Niazi, J. H. (2020). CdSe/CdS/ZnS nanocrystals decorated with Fe3O4 nanoparticles for point-of-care optomagnetic detection of cancer biomarker in serum. *Sensors and Actuators B: Chemical, 321*, 128431, https://doi.org/10.1016/j.snb.2020.128431.
31. Cheng, F., Su, L., & Qian, C. (2016). Circulating tumor DNA: a promising biomarker in the liquid biopsy of cancer. *Oncotarget, 7*(30), 48832–48841, https://doi.org/10.18632/oncotarget.9453.
32. Saha, S., Araf, Y., & Promon, S. K. (2022). Circulating tumor DNA in cancer diagnosis, monitoring, and prognosis. *Journal of the Egyptian National Cancer Institute, 34*(1), 8, https://doi.org/10.1186/s43046-022-00109-4.
33. Bartolomucci, A., Nobrega, M., Ferrier, T., Dickinson, K., Kaorey, N., Nadeau, A., et al. (2025). Circulating tumor DNA to monitor treatment response in solid tumors and advance precision oncology. *NPJ Precis Oncol, 9*(1), 84, https://doi.org/10.1038/s41698-025-00876-y.
34. Filis, P., Kyrochristos, I., Korakaki, E., Baltagiannis, E. G., Thanos, D., & Roukos, D. H. (2023). Longitudinal ctDNA profiling in precision oncology and immuno-oncology. *Drug Discov Today, 28*(4), 103540, https://doi.org/10.1016/j.drudis.2023.103540.
35. Das, J., Ivanov, I., Sargent, E. H., & Kelley, S. O. (2016). DNA Clutch Probes for Circulating Tumor DNA Analysis. *Journal of the American Chemical Society, 138*(34), 11009–11016, https://doi.org/10.1021/jacs.6b05679.
36. Pan, M., Wang, Z., Dai, Y., Yuan, R., & Wang, H. (2024). Al-Doped CuS Colloidal Nanocrystals as a Highly Efficient Electrochemiluminescence Emitter for the Ultrasensitive Detection of Circulating Tumor DNA. *Analytical Chemistry, 96*(38), 15430–15435.
37. Mishra, M., Ahmed, R., Das, D. K., Pramanik, D. D., Dash, S. K., & Pramanik, A. (2024). Recent Advancements in the Application of Circulating Tumor DNA as Biomarkers for Early Detection of Cancers. *ACS Biomaterials Science & Engineering, 10*(8), 4740–4756, https://doi.org/10.1021/acsbiomaterials.4c00606.
38. Becerra, A. Z., Probst, C. P., Tejani, M. A., Aquina, C. T., González, M. G., Hensley, B. J., et al. (2016). Evaluating the prognostic role of elevated preoperative carcinoembryonic antigen levels in colon cancer patients: results from the national cancer database. *Annals of surgical oncology, 23*, 1554–1561.
39. Jayanthi, V. S. A., Das, A. B., & Saxena, U. (2017). Recent advances in biosensor development for the detection of cancer biomarkers. *Biosensors and Bioelectronics, 91*, 15–23.

40. Tiernan, J., Perry, S., Verghese, E., West, N., Yeluri, S., Jayne, D., et al. (2013). Carcinoembryonic antigen is the preferred biomarker for in vivo colorectal cancer targeting. *British journal of cancer, 108*(3), 662–667.
41. Verberne, C., Wiggers, T., Grossmann, I., de Bock, G., & Vermeulen, K. (2016). Cost-effectiveness of a carcinoembryonic antigen (CEA) based follow-up programme for colorectal cancer (the CEA Watch trial). *Colorectal Disease, 18*(3), O91–O96.
42. Gao, Y., Song, P., Li, H., Jia, H., & Zhang, B. (2017). Elevated serum CEA levels are associated with the explosive progression of lung adenocarcinoma harboring EGFR mutations. *BMC cancer, 17*, 1–7.
43. Tran, D. T., Kim, N. H., & Lee, J. H. (2018). Cu-Au nanocrystals functionalized carbon nanotube arrays vertically grown on carbon spheres for highly sensitive detecting cancer biomarker. *Biosensors and Bioelectronics, 119*, 134–140.
44. Su, S., Han, X., Lu, Z., Liu, W., Zhu, D., Chao, J., et al. (2017). Facile synthesis of a MoS2–Prussian blue nanocube nanohybrid-based electrochemical sensing platform for hydrogen peroxide and carcinoembryonic antigen detection. *ACS Appl Mater Interfaces, 9*(14), 12773–12781.
45. Yang, Y., Liu, Q., Liu, Y., Cui, J., Liu, H., Wang, P., et al. (2017). A novel label-free electrochemical immunosensor based on functionalized nitrogen-doped graphene quantum dots for carcinoembryonic antigen detection. *Biosensors and Bioelectronics, 90*, 31–38.
46. Li, M., Li, J., Ding, X., He, M., & Cheng, S.-Y. (2010). microRNA and cancer. *The AAPS journal, 12*, 309–317.
47. Hayes, J., Peruzzi, P. P., & Lawler, S. (2014). MicroRNAs in cancer: biomarkers, functions and therapy. *Trends in molecular medicine, 20*(8), 460–469.
48. Wu, L., & Qu, X. (2015). Cancer biomarker detection: recent achievements and challenges. *Chemical Society Reviews, 44*(10), 2963–2997.
49. Gu, T., Li, Z., Ren, Z., Li, X., & Han, G. (2019). Rare-earth-doped upconversion nanocrystals embedded mesoporous silica nanoparticles for multiple microRNA detection. *Chemical Engineering Journal, 374*, 863–869.
50. Li, P., Wang, D., Hu, J., & Yang, X. (2022). The role of imaging in targeted delivery of nanomedicine for cancer therapy. *Advanced Drug Delivery Reviews, 189*, 114447.
51. Hussain, S., Mubeen, I., Ullah, N., Shah, S. S. U. D., Khan, B. A., Zahoor, M., et al. (2022). Modern diagnostic imaging technique applications and risk factors in the medical field: a review. *BioMed research international, 2022*(1), 5164970.
52. Shahbazi-Gahrouei, D., Khaniabadi, P. M., Khaniabadi, B. M., & Shahbazi-Gahrouei, S. (2019). Medical imaging modalities using nanoprobes for cancer diagnosis: A literature review on recent findings. *journal of research in medical sciences, 24*(1), 38.
53. Frangioni, J. V. (2008). New technologies for human cancer imaging. *Journal of clinical oncology, 26*(24), 4012–4021.
54. Hussain, T., & Nguyen, Q. T. (2014). Molecular imaging for cancer diagnosis and surgery. *Advanced Drug Delivery Reviews, 66*, 90–100.
55. James, M. L., & Gambhir, S. S. (2012). A molecular imaging primer: modalities, imaging agents, and applications. *Physiological reviews, 92*(2), 897–965.
56. Kircher, M. F., & Willmann, J. K. (2012). Molecular body imaging: MR imaging, CT, and US. part I. principles. *Radiology, 263*(3), 633–643.
57. Lai, L.-Y., Jiang, Y., Su, G.-P., Wu, M., Lu, X.-F., Fu, S.-Z., et al. (2021). Gadolinium-chelate functionalized magnetic CuFeSe2 ternary nanocrystals for T1-T2 dual MRI and CT imaging in vitro and in vivo. *Materials Research Express, 8*(4), 045001.
58. Kircher, M. F., & Willmann, J. K. (2012). Molecular body imaging: MR imaging, CT, and US. Part II. Applications. *Radiology, 264*(2), 349–368.

59. Key, J., & Leary, J. F. (2014). Nanoparticles for multimodal in vivo imaging in nanomedicine. *International journal of nanomedicine*, 711–726.
60. Sim, A. J., Kaza, E., Singer, L., & Rosenberg, S. A. (2020). A review of the role of MRI in diagnosis and treatment of early stage lung cancer. *Clinical and Translational Radiation Oncology, 24*, 16–22.
61. Rahman, M. (2023). Magnetic resonance imaging and iron-oxide nanoparticles in the era of personalized medicine. *Nanotheranostics, 7*(4), 424.
62. Cruz, L. J., Que, I., Aswendt, M., Chan, A., Hoehn, M., & Löwik, C. (2016). Targeted nanoparticles for the non-invasive detection of traumatic brain injury by optical imaging and fluorine magnetic resonance imaging. *Nano Research, 9*, 1276–1289.
63. Lapusan, R., Borlan, R., & Focsan, M. (2024). Advancing MRI with magnetic nanoparticles: a comprehensive review of translational research and clinical trials. *Nanoscale Advances*.
64. Jun, Y.-w., Huh, Y.-M., Choi, J.-s., Lee, J.-H., Song, H.-T., Kim, S., et al. (2005). Nanoscale size effect of magnetic nanocrystals and their utilization for cancer diagnosis via magnetic resonance imaging. *Journal of the American Chemical Society, 127*(16), 5732–5733.
65. Jia, Q., Ji, X., Wang, M., Wang, M., Zhang, S., He, L., et al. (2024). Photoelectric active copper/iron porphyrin-based metal–organic framework embedded with ferric oxide nanocrystals for photoelectrochemical aptasensing miRNA-141 and in vivo tumor magnetic resonance imaging. *Microchemical Journal, 204*, 111067.
66. Yang, G., Xia, J., Dai, X., Zhao, H., Gao, W., Ding, W., et al. (2024). A targeted multicrystalline manganese oxide as a tumor-selective nano-sized MRI contrast agent for early and accurate diagnosis of tumors. *International journal of nanomedicine*, 527–540.
67. Pelc, N. J. (2014). Recent and future directions in CT imaging. *Annals of biomedical engineering, 42*, 260–268.
68. Wu, Y., Sun, Y., Zhu, X., Liu, Q., Cao, T., Peng, J., et al. (2014). Lanthanide-based nanocrystals as dual-modal probes for SPECT and X-ray CT imaging. *Biomaterials, 35*(16), 4699–4705.
69. Pulumati, A., Pulumati, A., Dwarakanath, B. S., Verma, A., & Papineni, R. V. (2023). Technological advancements in cancer diagnostics: Improvements and limitations. *Cancer Reports, 6*(2), e1764.
70. Wang, Z., Chen, L., Huang, C., Huang, Y., & Jia, N. (2017). Albumin-mediated platinum nanocrystals for in vivo enhanced computed tomography imaging. *Journal of Materials Chemistry B, 5*(19), 3498–3510.
71. Paganin-Gioanni, A., Bellard, E., Paquereau, L., Ecochard, V., Golzio, M., & Teissié, J. (2010). Fluorescence imaging agents in cancerology. *Radiology and oncology, 44*(3), 142.
72. Lou, K.-L., Wang, P.-Y., Yang, R.-Q., Gao, Y.-Y., Tian, H.-N., Dang, Y.-Y., et al. (2022). Fabrication of tumor targeting rare-earth nanocrystals for real-time NIR-IIb fluorescence imaging-guided breast cancer precise surgery. *Nanomedicine: Nanotechnology, Biology and Medicine, 43*, 102555.
73. Frangioni, J. V. (2003). In vivo near-infrared fluorescence imaging. *Current opinion in chemical biology, 7*(5), 626–634.
74. Jenkins, R., Burdette, M. K., & Foulger, S. H. (2016). Mini-review: fluorescence imaging in cancer cells using dye-doped nanoparticles. *Rsc Advances, 6*(70), 65459-65474.
75. He, X., Gao, J., Gambhir, S. S., & Cheng, Z. (2010). Near-infrared fluorescent nanoprobes for cancer molecular imaging: status and challenges. *Trends in molecular medicine, 16*(12), 574–583.
76. Hu, G., Ning, J., Wu, T., Li, Y., Nie, Y., Lei, J., et al. (2024). A multifunctional cellulose nanocomposite with targeted fluorescence imaging and photothermal effects on breast cancer cells. *Cellulose, 31*(6), 3645–3656.

77. Bischof, J., Fletcher, G., Verkade, P., Kuntner, C., Fernandez-Rodriguez, J., Chaabane, L., et al. (2024). Multimodal bioimaging across disciplines and scales: challenges, opportunities and breaking down barriers. *npj Imaging, 2*(1), 5.
78. Fan, Y., He, A., Fan, M., Pei, Y., Chen, L., Liu, X., et al. (2025). In vivo tracking of nanoparticle metabolic pathways using 177Lu-labeled lanthanide-based nanocrystal via time-resolved and SPECT multimodal imaging☆. *Journal of Rare Earths*.
79. Jiang, X., Zhang, S., Ren, F., Chen, L., Zeng, J., Zhu, M., et al. (2017). Ultrasmall magnetic CuFeSe2 ternary nanocrystals for multimodal imaging guided photothermal therapy of cancer. *ACS nano, 11*(6), 5633–5645.
80. Chen, X., & Wong, S. T. (2014). Cancer theranostics: an introduction. In *Cancer Theranostics* (pp. 3–8): Elsevier.
81. Sumer, B., & Gao, J. (2008). Theranostic nanomedicine for cancer. *Nanomedicine, 3*(2), 137–140.
82. Ahmed, N., Fessi, H., & Elaissari, A. (2012). Theranostic applications of nanoparticles in cancer. *Drug Discov Today, 17*(17–18), 928–934.
83. Conte, M., Carofiglio, M., Vander Pol, R. S., Wood, A., Hernandez, N., Joubert, A., et al. (2025). Acoustically Driven Hybrid Nanocrystals for In Vivo Pancreatic Cancer Treatment. *ACS Appl Mater Interfaces, 17*(8), 11873–11887.
84. Muller, M., Haghnejad, V., Schaefer, M., Gauchotte, G., Caron, B., Peyrin-Biroulet, L., et al. (2022). The immune landscape of human pancreatic ductal carcinoma: key players, clinical implications, and challenges. *Cancers (Basel), 14*(4), 995.
85. Geyer, M., Gaul, L.-M., DAgosto, S. L., Corbo, V., & Queiroz, K. (2023). The tumor stroma influences immune cell distribution and recruitment in a PDAC-on-a-chip model. *Frontiers in Immunology, 14*, 1155085.
86. Canta, M., & Cauda, V. (2020). The investigation of the parameters affecting the ZnO nanoparticle cytotoxicity behaviour: a tutorial review. *Biomaterials science, 8*(22), 6157–6174.
87. George, S., Pokhrel, S., Xia, T., Gilbert, B., Ji, Z., Schowalter, M., et al. (2010). Use of a rapid cytotoxicity screening approach to engineer a safer zinc oxide nanoparticle through iron doping. *ACS nano, 4*(1), 15–29.
88. Xia, T., Zhao, Y., Sager, T., George, S., Pokhrel, S., Li, N., et al. (2011). Decreased dissolution of ZnO by iron doping yields nanoparticles with reduced toxicity in the rodent lung and zebrafish embryos. *ACS nano, 5*(2), 1223–1235.
89. Xu, C., Nam, J., Hong, H., Xu, Y., & Moon, J. J. (2019). Positron emission tomography-guided photodynamic therapy with biodegradable mesoporous silica nanoparticles for personalized cancer immunotherapy. *ACS nano, 13*(10), 12148–12161.
90. Cao, W., Chen, H.-D., Yu, Y.-W., Li, N., & Chen, W.-Q. (2021). Changing profiles of cancer burden worldwide and in China: a secondary analysis of the global cancer statistics 2020. *Chinese medical journal, 134*(7), 783–791.
91. Iranshahy, M., Rezaee, R., & Karimi, G. (2019). Hepatoprotective activity of metformin: a new mission for an old drug? *European journal of pharmacology, 850*, 1–7.
92. Anwanwan, D., Singh, S. K., Singh, S., Saikam, V., & Singh, R. (2020). Challenges in liver cancer and possible treatment approaches. *Biochimica et biophysica acta (BBA)-Reviews on cancer, 1873*(1), 188314.
93. Xing, L., Yang, X., Bai, J., Zhong, C., Cai, J., Dan, Q., et al. (2025). Use of UMFNPs/Ce6@MBs in multimodal imaging-guided sono-photodynamic combination therapy for hepatocellular carcinoma. *Biomaterials science, 13*(1), 179–192.
94. Siegel, R. L., Miller, K. D., Fuchs, H. E., & Jemal, A. (2022). Cancer statistics, 2022. *CA: a cancer journal for clinicians, 72*(1), 7–33.

95. Zeng, L., Gowda, B. H. J., Ahmed, M. G., Abourehab, M. A. S., Chen, Z.-S., Zhang, C., et al. (2023). Advancements in nanoparticle-based treatment approaches for skin cancer therapy. *Molecular Cancer, 22*(1), 10, https://doi.org/10.1186/s12943-022-01708-4.
96. Hasan, N., Nadaf, A., Imran, M., Jiba, U., Sheikh, A., Almalki, W. H., et al. (2023). Skin cancer: understanding the journey of transformation from conventional to advanced treatment approaches. *Molecular Cancer, 22*(1), 168, https://doi.org/10.1186/s12943-023-01854-3.
97. Borlan, R., Tudor, M., Soritau, O., Florea, A., Pall, E., Pop, B., et al. (2024). Dual-modal near-infrared organic nanoparticles: integrating mild hyperthermia phototherapy with fluorescence imaging. *International journal of nanomedicine*, 9071–9090.
98. Bian, W., Wang, Y., Pan, Z., Chen, N., Li, X., Wong, W.-L., et al. (2021). Review of Functionalized Nanomaterials for Photothermal Therapy of Cancers. *ACS Applied Nano Materials, 4*(11), 11353–11385, https://doi.org/10.1021/acsanm.1c01903.
99. Zhao, L., Zhang, X., Wang, X., Guan, X., Zhang, W., & Ma, J. (2021). Recent advances in selective photothermal therapy of tumor. *Journal of Nanobiotechnology, 19*(1), 335, https://doi.org/10.1186/s12951-021-01080-3.
100. Nomura, S., Morimoto, Y., Tsujimoto, H., Arake, M., Harada, M., Saitoh, D., et al. (2020). Highly reliable, targeted photothermal cancer therapy combined with thermal dosimetry using a near-infrared absorbent. *Scientific Reports, 10*(1), 9765, https://doi.org/10.1038/s41598-020-66646-x.
101. Morrow, M. (2025). Sentinel-Lymph-Node Biopsy in Early-Stage Breast Cancer - Is It Obsolete? *N Engl J Med, 392*(11), 1134–1136, https://doi.org/10.1056/NEJMe2414899.
102. Matsuo, K., Klar, M., Nusbaum, D. J., Hasanov, M. F., Vallejo, A., Ciesielski, K. M., et al. (2022). Utilization and Outcomes of Sentinel Lymph Node Biopsy for Early Endometrial Cancer. *Obstet Gynecol, 139*(5), 809–820, https://doi.org/10.1097/aog.0000000000004733.
103. Tang, D., Cui, M., Wang, B., Liang, G., Zhang, H., & Xiao, H. (2024). Nanoparticles destabilizing the cell membranes triggered by NIR light for cancer imaging and photo-immunotherapy. *Nature Communications, 15*(1), 6026, https://doi.org/10.1038/s41467-024-50020-w.
104. Yang, Z., Zhang, Z., Sun, Y., Lei, Z., Wang, D., Ma, H., et al. (2021). Incorporating spin-orbit coupling promoted functional group into an enhanced electron D-A system: A useful designing concept for fabricating efficient photosensitizer and imaging-guided photodynamic therapy. *Biomaterials, 275*, 120934, https://doi.org/10.1016/j.biomaterials.2021.120934.
105. Zhang, Y. H., Li, X., Huang, L., Kim, H. S., An, J., Lan, M., et al. (2020). AIE based GSH activatable photosensitizer for imaging-guided photodynamic therapy. *Chem Commun (Camb), 56*(71), 10317–10320, https://doi.org/10.1039/d0cc02045a.
106. Liu, T., Liu, W., Zhang, M., Yu, W., Gao, F., Li, C., et al. (2018). Ferrous-Supply-Regeneration Nanoengineering for Cancer-Cell-Specific Ferroptosis in Combination with Imaging-Guided Photodynamic Therapy. *ACS nano, 12*(12), 12181–12192, https://doi.org/10.1021/acsnano.8b05860.
107. Lin, W., Sun, T., Xie, Z., Gu, J., & Jing, X. (2016). A dual-responsive nanocapsule via disulfide-induced self-assembly for therapeutic agent delivery. *Chem Sci, 7*(3), 1846–1852, https://doi.org/10.1039/c5sc03707g.
108. Zhang, Q., Cai, Y., Li, Q. Y., Hao, L. N., Ma, Z., Wang, X. J., et al. (2017). Targeted Delivery of a Mannose-Conjugated BODIPY Photosensitizer by Nanomicelles for Photodynamic Breast Cancer Therapy. *Chemistry, 23*(57), 14307–14315, https://doi.org/10.1002/chem.201702935.

109. Zhang, J., Huang, H., Xue, L., Zhong, L., Ge, W., Song, X., et al. (2020). On-demand drug release nanoplatform based on fluorinated aza-BODIPY for imaging-guided chemo-phototherapy. *Biomaterials, 256*, 120211, https://doi.org/10.1016/j.biomaterials.2020.120211.
110. Mai, D. K., Kim, C., Lee, J., Vales, T. P., Badon, I. W., De, K., et al. (2022). BODIPY nanoparticles functionalized with lactose for cancer-targeted and fluorescence imaging-guided photodynamic therapy. *Scientific Reports, 12*(1), 2541, https://doi.org/10.1038/s41598-022-06000-5.

# Toxicity, Clinical Studies of Nanocrystals, Conclusion and Future Scope

Nanotechnology has undoubtedly transformed the field of cancer diagnosis and therapy owing to the large surface area with high penetration power to invade the tumour microenvironment [1], greater bioavailability and being amenable to surface modification with drugs, antibodies, nucleic acids etc. to specifically target the cancer cells [2, 3]. The increasing popularity of nanocrystals in cancer theranostics is due to the simple fact that nanoparticles can be used in combination with detection as well as therapeutic agents to provide a more patient-friendly platform, combining detection, therapy and overcoming drug-resistance in a single unit, while eliminating the individual toxicity and enhancing patient convenience [4].

## 7.1 Toxicity of Nanocrystals

The major drawback of chemotherapy medicines is their widespread systemic toxicity and low therapeutic efficacy [5]. Various nanocrystal-drug conjugates are reported to reduce the unwanted toxicity of chemotherapy drugs and ensure better localization [6]. Recent years have evidenced extensive techniques are used to prepare diverse categories of nanocrystals both organic and inorganic, like metal-ion based, liposome based, protein based, carbon nanotubes and quantum dots, with unique properties that can combine the diagnosis (imaging) of cancer cells and target them for delivering therapeutic outcome simultaneously [4]. For example, gold and silver possess surface plasmon resonance (SPR) that can be modulated accordingly, making them important candidates for theranostics applications [7, 8]. However, the toxicity of the nanocrystals used in cancer theranostics is a crucial area of consideration while implementing these nanocrystals in treating cancer patients in real-world settings. It has been observed that even after notable success in the cell and animal models, theranostic nanocrystals demonstrate significant toxicity in human patients. Several advanced effects disable the functionality of the nanocrystals, thus failing to prove their efficacy when tested in clinical trials. In various studies, the occurrence of adverse side effects on the human subjects have led to patient withdrawal or termination of the clinical trial even before completion.

In 2007, a multicenter clinical study was conducted in the United States, employing patients with kidney cancer who has earlier shown disease progression after being treated with the FDA approved anti-angiogenic drug, sunitinib malate. In this Phase II human trial, the patients were treated with 2-methoxyestradiol nanocrystals (marketed as Panzem) alone and in co-treatment with sunitinib malate. The patient outcomes were highly unsatisfactory, with no improvement in tumour metastasis. The dose specified for the study proved to be toxic to the patients, giving rise to adverse effects like skin irritation, grade 3 increment in liver enzymes like ALT and AST, fatigue and loss of appetite. Grade 3 dyspnea was found in one patient. Owing to poor tolerance, 35% of the patients resigned from the study and trial was terminated early in 2009. Till then, modified analogues of Panzem NCD are under development but none has reached the stage of clinical study [9]. Some instances of nanocrystal toxicity and how modern research is coping up with these limitations are discussed below.

### 7.1.1 Hydrophilic Nanocrystals

One of approaches to combat the off-target toxicity of nanocrystals used in cancer theranostics includes coating them with hydrophilic materials like polyethylene glycol (PEG), folate, aptamers, transferrin, hyaluronic acid and antibodies. This not only makes the nanosystem hydrophilic, but also helps in specific recognition and accumulation in cancer cells [8]. Metal oxide like Zinc-oxide is well known for its genotoxicity, the fact that is widely explored in anti-cancer therapy. Recently, ZnO nanocrystals have been surface modified by addition of functional groups like oleic acid, carboxylate and PEG to enhance their hydrophilicity surface area, biocompatibility, functionality and biodegradability leading to reduction in cytotoxicity [10].

## 7.1.2 Organic Nanocrystals

Organic nanocrystals appear significantly promising for cancer theranostics due to their ability of improved drug delivery, better penetration and lower side effects compared to traditional nanoparticles. This is because organic nanocrystals are biodegradable, non-toxic stable in biological fluids and can be modified to make responsive to electromagnetic stimuli [11]. Some of the commonly used organic nanocrystals include polymers, dendrimers, micelles, liposomes, chitosan, silk fibroin and ferritin [12]. The toxicity of these nanocrystals varies greatly on the nature of organic molecule used during synthesis, size, shape, surface modifications, dosage and route of administration. Modern research has focussed in the optimization of design and synthesis of the organic nanocrystals to enhance their biocompatibility and safety profile, minimize their toxic side effects so as to ensure fruitful translation to clinical purpose.

## 7.1.3 Lipid-Based Nanoparticles

Liposomal and lipid nanosystems belong to a specific group of organic nanoparticles which are extensively used to deliver theranostic agents due to their flexibility to accommodate both hydrophilic and hydrophobic molecules [13]. Various studies have explored lipid carriers to deliver diagnostic contrast agents based on $^{14}C$ [14], $^{64}Cu$ [15], quantum dots (QDs), gadolinium (Gd) [16] etc. They are biodegradable and their surfaces can be modified according to the therapeutic goal to specifically target the cancer cells [13]. This reduces the chances of undesired toxicity and are hence are recently explored in clinical trials for cancer patients [17, 18]. Lin et al. presented a unique platform for real-time monitoring of drug delivery in a prostate tumour model using dye- and siRNA-loaded lipid nanoparticles (LNPs) [19]. Theranostic iron oxide nanocrystals with porphyrin-conjugated lipid coat (Fe3O4@PGLNPs) showed significant photodynamic effects against HT-29 cancer cell line [20].

## 7.1.4 Bioinspired Nanocrystals

A special group of organic nanocrystals are bioinspired nanoparticles, that are based on molecules naturally synthesized in the biological system. Bioinspired nanocrystals being derived from naturally occurring products like proteins, lipids, virus particles, polymers like chitosan, silk etc., are comparatively biocompatible than synthesized nanoparticles and hence offers negligible toxicity [21]. They range from 1 to 100 nm in diameter and demonstrate definite physiochemical behaviour that allow them to enable more effective interactions with the tumour cells [22]. However, after extraction from the biological source, they need to be purified and optimization of parameters for their designing needs to carefully done before diagnosis and therapeutic agents are incorporated into them so as to have minimal toxic effects, when used in clinical settings.

Cellulose nanoparticles (CNC NPs) show a wide range of physical and chemical features, that making them attractive target in drug delivery and theranostics applications [23, 24]. Studies suggest that the definitive needle-like or rod shape of the cellulose nanocrystals can easily penetrate the lung vasculature and disrupt the development of new blood vessels in metastatic lung tumours [25]. Imlimthan et al. developed a novel treatment for lung metastatic melanoma using cellulose nanocrystals that were implemented to deliver radioactive drug ($^{177}$Lu) and an anti-cancer drug (vemurafenib) directly to the tumours. The nanosystem offered promising results in lung melanoma model [26]. Unfortunately, various studies suggest that cellulose nanocrystals can evoke immunogenic and inflammatory responses in animal body, which needs proper management before they are translated for clinical purpose [27] (Fig. 7.1).

Albumin-bound paclitaxel, (marketed as Abraxane), represents promising advancement in the treatment of metastatic breast cancer. Traditional taxanes, a standard chemotherapy for this disease, often rely on solvents in their formulations to ensure drug solubility. However, these solvents are associated with significant toxicities, limiting the tolerability and potentially the efficacy of the treatment. To overcome this challenge, a solvent-free

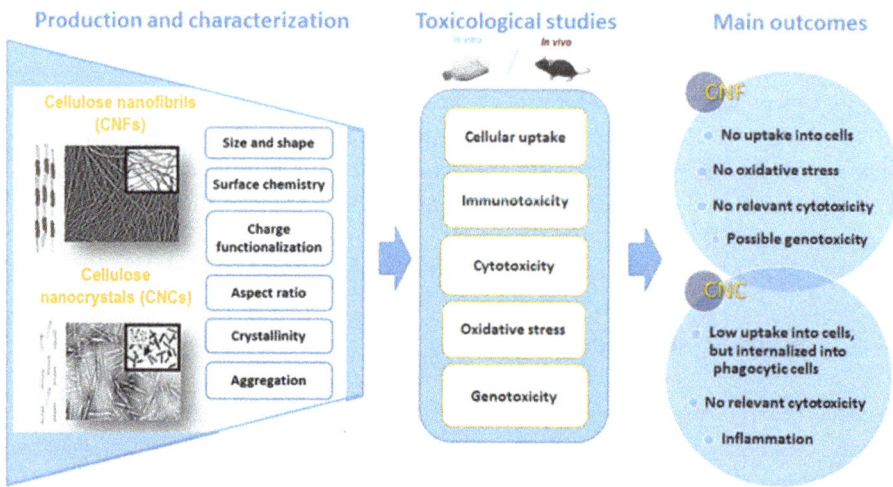

**Fig. 7.1** Schematic representation highlighting the toxic outcomes of cellulose nanocrystals [27]

## 7.1 Toxicity of Nanocrystals

formulation of paclitaxel of nearly 130 nm has been developed using human albumin nanoparticles. By binding paclitaxel to albumin, a naturally occurring protein in the blood, the drug is observed to reach more efficiently to the tumour site, potentially enhancing drug delivery and reducing systemic exposure to the toxic solvents. The FDA approval of nab-paclitaxel underscores its clinical significance as a next-generation taxane that mitigates solvent-related toxicities while effectively targeting metastatic breast cancer [28].

### 7.1.5 Metal–Organic Framework

Traditional chemotherapy medicines are known for causing damage to normal healthy tissues of the body. Metal–organic frameworks (MOFs) are a diverse category of nanosystem that includes metals (mainly elements of d and f block) conjugated with organic linkers [29] to form a porous structure that can encapsulate the therapeutic or imaging agent used in cancer cell elimination. The encapsulating framework prevents off-target release of therapeutic agent and ensure sustained release of it. They provide the provision for tuning their surface with tumour recognizing ligands that ensures therapeutic outcome only at the specific tumour site, diminishing systemic toxicity [30]. MOFs provide a suitable platform for implementing radiation therapy [31], chemotherapy and photodynamic therapy (PTD) through guidance obtained by simultaneous imaging by the diagnostic agent that is co-delivered within the same system [32, 33].

Wang et al. created a Zn-based MOF using TATAT ligands with high drug loading capacity and exerted sustained delivery of anticancer agent, 5-fluorouracil (5-FU) for 1 week [34]. In another study, a MOF nanocomposite was developed that executed fluorescent based MRI technique to detect the cancer cells and deliver 5-FU at the target site [35]. Liu et al., manufactured UiO-66-$NH_2$ nanoparticles modified with folic acid (FA) and the fluorescent imaging agent 5-carboxyfluorescein (5-FAM) to create a multifaceted theranostic system, demonstrated tumour detection and enhanced antitumour efficacy in vivo due to sustained drug release [36]. In a separate study, Cherkasov et al. developed an MOF functionalized with antibodies that selectively target and absorb HER2/neu-positive cancer cells [37].

### 7.1.6 Quantum Dots (QD)

QD-nanoparticle hybridization holds potential significance for creating multifunctional nanomedicines in cancer theranostics. Gold nanoparticle (AuNP) and quantum dot (QD) hybrids have theranostic application in cancer. Chen et al. developed zinc oxide QDs combined with camptothecin-containing AuNPs, where AuNPs facilitate photothermal tumor destruction [38]. Another approach combines paramagnetic Gd ions with CuInS/ZnS QDs for both fluorescence and magnetic resonance-based imaging [39]. Yang et al. created Gd-doped zinc sulphide QDs in lipid vesicles, that produced fluorescence and were stable in the absence of Cadmium. To prevent fluorescence quenching, $Fe_3O_4$ nanoparticles were removed away from graphene-CdTe QDs by a $SiO_2$ barrier, allowing for 5-Fluorouracil loading for hepatoma treatment [40]. However, Quantum dots (QDs) exhibit several mechanisms of toxicity, including unwanted immune responses, apoptosis and necrosis of cells, and genotoxicity, causing damage to genetic material. These effects are often linked to the leeching of heavy metals from the QDs, generating oxidative stress. The small size of QDs also allows them ton react with cellular components and organelles, potentially disrupting normal functions. Strategies like coating QDs with biocompatible agents are being explored to mitigate these toxic effects [41].

Quantum dots (QD) show properties like photoluminescence and high values for molar extinction coefficient and are much more efficient than conventional dyes used for imaging, that makes harboured for detection of cancer cells and delivering the therapeutic intervention [42]. Unfortunately, there have reports for non-targeted QD toxicity and oxidative stress, particularly those containing Cd ions [43], that acts as a major barrier for their clinical translation [44]. Another significant challenge lies in the potential for off-target accumulation of QDs in the Reticular endothelial system, that reduces the probability and overall functionality of these theranostic agents in selectively binding to the intended neoplastic site [45]. Thus, to ensure non-toxic tumour imaging and treatment, QDs are coated with biomaterials like lipids, proteins and polysaccharides that helps in reducing the systemic toxicity [46].

One of the most popularly explored polysaccharides used for this purpose is chitosan. To further eliminate the toxicity of chitosan, Bwatanglang et al. developed Mn-doped ZnS QDs functionalized with folic acid to ensure targeted drug delivery for cancer theranostics [47]. In this approach, the imaging functionality of Mn:ZnS QDs were integrated within the same system. The nanocomposite demonstrated excellent biocompatibility on healthy (MCF-10) and cancerous breast cells (MCF-7) even at a high concentration. Moreover, folic acid on the surface of QDs could recognize its receptors present on the cancer cells to enable their detection through enhanced fluorescence. Graphene QDs were previously identified to be nontoxic and safe to healthy cells [48]. But there are several reports of composites of GO enhancing the ROS production and producing toxicity to biological systems [49]. Therefore, significant in vivo studies need to be performed to confirm its safety and toxicity profile before they can be implemented in cancer theranostics.

## 7.1.7 Carbon Dots (CD) and Carbon-Based Nanocrystals

Carbon dots (CD) are widely used in in cancer treatment delivering therapeutic agents for chemotherapy, radiotherapy, photothermal therapy (PTT) [50], photodynamic therapy (PDT) and gene therapy. They are small in size, demonstrates high permeability and retention in the cancer cells and can easily eliminated by the urinary system, thus reducing toxicity [51, 52]. They can penetrate the stem cells without hampering their differentiation [53]. It has been verified that attachment of specific ligands on the CDs can allow more specific targeting and internalisation of therapeutic agent on cancerous cells (MDAMB and A-549) as compared to healthy control (MDCK) cells[54, 55]. This is why CD formulations with photosensitive agents like photoporphyrin and zinc phthalocyanine are investigated for NIR light mediated photodynamic therapy through ROS production [56–58].

Fullerene is a potential molecule used in cancer theranostics owing to its flexible physio-chemical properties [59]. It can not only act as free-radical scavenger but can also be conjugated with metal compounds that can exploited for cancer detection through MRI, X-ray imaging or radio imaging [60]. However, the major drawback of this compound is its poor water solubility and evidences of intrinsic toxicity. Modern researchers have hence focussed on modifying the base compound with hydrophilic and biocompatible moieties to develop a more useful compound, referred to as the biocompatible fullerene [61].

Serda et al. developed a fullerene derivative based on carbon-60 modified with glucosamine to combat pancreatic cancer. This novel drug preferentially accumulated in the pancreatic stellate cells, likely due to the increased glucose metabolism in tumours [62]. In another approach, the fullerene conjugate (C60-Dex-NH$_2$) was used to target cancer cells through RNA interference (RNAi) technology, delivering siRNAs [63].

## 7.1.8 Inorganic Nanocrystals

Inorganic nanoparticles, distinguished by their exceptional physicochemical attributes encompassing magnetic, thermal, optical, and catalytic properties, alongside their versatile functionalities in bioimaging, targeted delivery, and controlled therapeutic release facilitated by surface engineering or dopant incorporation, have been identified as a suitable platform in theranostic purpose in cancer research. Nevertheless, their inherent resistance to degradation and excretion within biological systems engenders protracted residence times, potentially culminating in adverse sequelae such as inflammatory responses and tissue granuloma formation, thereby impeding their clinical translation. Consequently, the advent of biodegradable inorganic nanomaterials represents a pivotal advancement, holding immense promise for their safe and efficacious deployment in biomedical applications [64].

Silica nanoparticles have been widely explored in biomedical applications, both in diagnostic [65] and drug delivery [66] purposes because of their biocompatibility and biodegradable properties, which aids their easy elimination by the renal system. Several research have been conducted to enhance the biodegration of the silica nanocrystals in vivo. In one study, chitosan was conjugated with mesoporous silica nanoparticles to generate degradable nanosystem delivering therapeutic drugs specifically to the breast cancer tissues. It was found that the nanocarrier system demonstrated excellent biocompatibility in the living system [67].

Iron-oxide nanocrystals possess paramagnetic properties which makes them suitable materials to be used as MRI contrast agents in theranostic purposes. It is poorly soluble in body fluids and have restricted transport and bioavailability. Gu et al. developed a PEGylated form of iron oxide nanocrystals with surface functionalised via oleic acid. The nanocrystals proved well penetration efficacy to the remote tissues of the body, but lacked clearance and biodegradation, thus increasing the chances of toxic accumulation in vivo [68].

Among the inorganic nanocrystals, silver nanocrystals show promising scope in cancer theranostics. Traditional method of silver nanoparticles (AgNPs) was mostly chemical, as it produced high yield and easy to execute. However, the growing evidences of toxicity due to chemical synthesis [69, 70] made the biochemists to shift their focus to an eco-friendlier 'green' approach to manufacture AgNPs from various biological sources [71]. Padinjarathil et al. prepared Ag nanocrystals from galactomannan [72] whereas AgNPs synthesized by Oves et al. from the roots of *Phoenix dactylifera* [73] demonstrated delicate anticancer efficacy in arresting the cell cycle of cancer cells at sub-G1 and S phase. Biocompatible AgNPs synthesized from the latex extract of *Calotropis gigantean* proved to selectively destroy the lymphoblastic leukaemia and ascites tumour EAC cell lines by initiating DNA damage through oxidative stress and apoptosis and prevents angiogenesis, while remaining non-toxic to human and mouse lymphocytes [74] In another study, Dinparvar et al. prepared AgNPs using the *Cuminum cyminum* seed extracts that evidenced excellent hostility against human breast cancer cells (MCF-7) and AU565 cancer cell line and were comparably less toxic than AgNPs synthesized chemically [75].

Copper-based nanocrystals (CuO, $Cu_2O$, $Cu_2S$, CuS, $Cu_2Se$ and CuSe) have garnered significant interest within the scientific community owing to their inherent biocompatibility and distinctive physicochemical characteristics [76]. Zhao et al. performed a significant work by developing quantum dots of silver-copper sulfide ($Ag_{2-x}Cu_xS$) within an integrated theranostic nanomedicine platform for photothermal therapy (PTT) to be performed using a low-power 635 nm laser. Furthermore, the study demonstrated the absence of long-term toxicity associated with these materials [77].

Thus, the main goal of using nanocrystals in cancer theranostics is to develop smarter nanomaterials react specifically to the tumour microenvironment with no residual toxicity towards the healthy body tissues [78].

## 7.2 Clinical Studies of Nanocrystals

Considerable research is being performed in the field of nanocrystal development for cancer theranostics. Scientists strive to generate novel nanomaterials that can serve the purpose of both the diagnosis and delivering therapy in a single unit. A lot of these materials get validated by their in vitro effects on the cancer cell lines, or through in vivo studies on rodents. However, a major gap is apprehended when these nanomedicines are tested for their efficacy on human patients. This is because the human physiology, inspite of its similarity to species like mice and rats, offers a much more complex scenario with diverse variety of cross-talk between diverse biomolecules and signalling pathways, that often restrict the clinical success of these nanoproducts. A major challenge in failure of nanocrystals for biomedical applications is the host-immune system. Therapies that provide positive outcomes in the pre-clinical studies are found to behave in a completely different manner when introduced in the human body. This gives rise to unwanted immune reactions, allergies, toxic side-effects and rejection of the theranostic intervention. Therefore, there is a necessary need to undergo clinical trials of the nanocrystals proposed in cancer theranostics before they receive FDA approval. The following table summarizes the outcomes of various clinical trials all over the world employing nanocrystals in cancer diagnosis and therapy (Table 7.1).

**Table 7.1** Clinical trials of nanocrystals used in cancer theranostics

| Sl. no. | Name of the nanocrystal | Clinical trial stage and ID | Application | Patient outcome | References |
|---|---|---|---|---|---|
| 1 | Panzem® (2-methoxyestradiol) | NCT00400348 (completed phase II trial) | Ovarian cancer | 50% of the patients demonstrated stable disease symptoms, where there was no further progression in the disease. Although the treatment was well tolerated, some adverse events like nausea, fatigue, diarrhoea and neuropathy was observed | [79] |
| 2 | Panzem® (2-methoxyestradiol) | NCT00306618 (completed phase II trial) | Glioblastoma | No positive patient outcomes are known till date | https://clinicaltrials.gov/study/NCT00306618?cond=Cancer&intr=nanocrystal&rank=2 |
| 3 | Panzem NCD in combination with fixed-dose temozolomide | NCT00481455 (completed phase II trial) | Recurrent glioblastoma Multiforme (GBM) | No positive patient outcomes are known till date | https://clinicaltrials.gov/study/NCT00481455?cond=Cancer&intr=nanocrystal&rank=5 |

(continued)

## 7.2 Clinical Studies of Nanocrystals

**Table 7.1** (continued)

| Sl. no. | Name of the nanocrystal | Clinical trial stage and ID | Application | Patient outcome | References |
|---|---|---|---|---|---|
| 4 | Panzem nanocrystal colloidal dispersion (NCD) in combination with anti-VEGF antibody Avastin (bevacizumab) | NCT00328497 (completed phase II trial) | Advanced or metastatic carcinoid tumors | The nanocrystal-drug therapy was well tolerated with a median progression free survival duration of 11.3 months | https://clinicaltrials.gov/study/NCT00328497?cond=Cancer&intr=nanocrystal&rank=3 |
| 5 | Panzem NCD | NCT00394810 (completed phase II trial) | Metastatic, androgen-independent prostate cancer | Anticancer activity was observed at a dose of 1200 mg/day for 4 weeks. Increase in liver transaminase activity and deep venous thromboses were the side-effects observed in 2 out of the 33 male patients enrolled | [80] |
| 6 | Panzem NCD combined with sunitinib malate | NCT00444314 (completed phase II trial) | Metastatic renal cell carcinoma progressing on Sunitinib Malate | No significant recovery of the patients was seen. Anti-tumour efficacy was mild. The study was terminated due to poor tolerance | [9] |

(continued)

Table 7.1 (continued)

| Sl. no. | Name of the nanocrystal | Clinical trial stage and ID | Application | Patient outcome | References |
|---|---|---|---|---|---|
| 7 | Semapimod nanocrystals (CNI-1493) in combination with Interleukin-2 | Completed phase I trial | Cancer patients | Reduced production of TNF-α involved in inflammation-induced cancer development. The drug was well-tolerated with few side effects such as phlebitis at the site of injection, hypotension | [81] |
| 8 | Theralux™ (thymectacin nanocrystal) | Phase I/II clinical trial (ongoing) | Photodynamic therapy in patients with non-Hodgkin's lymphoma, colon cancer | Patient outcomes are yet to be known | [82] |
| 9 | Abraxane (paclitaxel bound to albumin) | NCT00583349 (completed phase II trial) | Urinary bladder cancer with previous treatment with BCG | Out of 28 patients, one-fourth of them remained cancer free with promising survival rates (upto 91%) | [83] |
| 10 | Albumin-bound paclitaxel (ABI-007) | Completed phase III trial | Metastatic breast cancer | ABI-007 proved to be highly effective and demonstrated better safety profile as compared to standard paclitaxel in the patient group. However, ABI-007 treatment induced grade 3 neuropathy, that was easily managed | [84] |

(continued)

7.2 Clinical Studies of Nanocrystals 151

Table 7.1 (continued)

| Sl. no. | Name of the nanocrystal | Clinical trial stage and ID | Application | Patient outcome | References |
|---|---|---|---|---|---|
| 11 | Laser based immunotherapy with Indocyanine green (ICG) and N-dihydro-galacto-chitosan (GC) | NCT03202446 (phase III ongoing) | Metastatic breast cancer melanoma | The treatment eliminated the metastatic cancer cells in the patient population in Phase II trials with a clinical response rate of 75% | [85] |
| 12 | MBP-426 | NCT00355888 (phase I completed) | Metastatic solid tumours | MBP-426 was safe and showed reduction in tumour volume in 2 of the 39 patients. 15 of them demonstrated no further progression of the tumour following the treatment. Phase I/II trial (NCT00964080) was performed thereafter to evaluate the safety and utility of the nanocrystal used along with 5-FU/leucovorin (LV) in patients with alimentary canal carcinoma | [86] |

(continued)

**Table 7.1** (continued)

| Sl. no. | Name of the nanocrystal | Clinical trial stage and ID | Application | Patient outcome | References |
|---|---|---|---|---|---|
| 13 | TNF-bound colloidal gold nanocrystals silica–gold nanoparticles (NCT01270139) | NCT00356980 (phase I completed) | Advanced solid organ malignancies | Gold conjugation enhanced the distribution of TNF in patients and uptake in the tumour tissues. After its positive results in terms of safety and tolerance, the intervention is signed on 2020 to be carried to Phase II trials by Cytimmune company | [87] |
| 14 | Cornell dots (C dots) | NCT02106598 (phase II ongoing) | Real tumour tracing in melanoma patients for theranostic purpose | I-cRGDY–PEG–C dot consists of the fluorescent dye Cy5 and was significantly uptaken in the cancer tissue, enabling detection and therapy. The nanoparticles were well tolerated | [88] |
| 15 | BIND-014, a docetaxel nanoparticle | NCT01812746 (phase II completed) | Targeting the antigens specific for prostate cancer | Prostate-cancer specific antigens were reduced in the patients. Adverse side effects included fatigue, nausea and neuropathy | [89] |

(continued)

## 7.2 Clinical Studies of Nanocrystals

**Table 7.1** (continued)

| Sl. no. | Name of the nanocrystal | Clinical trial stage and ID | Application | Patient outcome | References |
|---|---|---|---|---|---|
| 16 | CINOVA: CPC634 (nanoparticulate docetaxel) | NCT03742713 (completed phase II trials) | Patients suffering from platinum resistant ovarian cancer | The study was stopped before completion due to poor efficacy and various adverse gastrointestinal side-effects, fatigue, hypertension | [90] |
| 17 | TKM-080.301 | NCT01437007 (phase I completed) | Advanced Liver cancer | 50% of a total of 39 subjects were observed to have stable disease. 2 subjects developed thrombocytopenia | [91] |
| 18 | NLG207 (formerly CRLX101) nanoparticle-bound and released camptothecin | NCT00333502 (phase II completed) | To study the release of camptothecin, a topoisomerase inhibitor in plasma of prostate cancer patients | Significant increase in camptothecin in the blood of the patients was observed | [92] |
| 19 | AGuIX nanocrystal in combination with radiochemotherapy and temozolomide | NCT04881032 (phase I/II study-ongoing) | Patients with newly diagnosed glioblastoma | The study is yet to be completed | [93] |
| 20 | Nafnium oxide (HfO$_2$) nanoparticle NBTXR3 activated by radiotherapy | NCT04505267 (phase II/III study completed) | Patients with locally advanced soft-tissue sarcoma | Positive clinical outcomes were found in 16% of the patients enrolled. Side effects included pain due to multiple injections, hypotension, skin damage following radiation | [94] |

## 7.3 Conclusion

Recent years have evidenced great progress in the field of nanotechnology for developing advanced materials for cancer theranostics. Nanomedicines come with the advantage of low particle size, high drug loading, greater surface area and amenable surfaces that increases the distribution of the employed drugs in the body. These nanoscale particles can easily invade the biological barriers and reach the body tissues, making them attractive targets for researchers working in cancer theranostics. Nanoparticles are widely explored to treat almost all types of cancers in the human body, such as glioblastoma, bone cancer, lung cancer, bladder cancer, prostate cancer, thyroid cancer, breast cancer and cancer in the digestive system (oesophagus, liver, pancreas and colon). Various contrast agents are formulated into nanosystem that serve cancer detection through imaging techniques like PET, CT, MRI, FI, biosensing etc. (Fig. 7.2).

Nanocrystals are colloidal systems, where particle size is reduced to nanoscale range and has been revolutionary in enhancing the bioavailability of drugs used in cancer theranostics. Poorly soluble oral drugs used as imaging agents or for therapeutic purpose pose

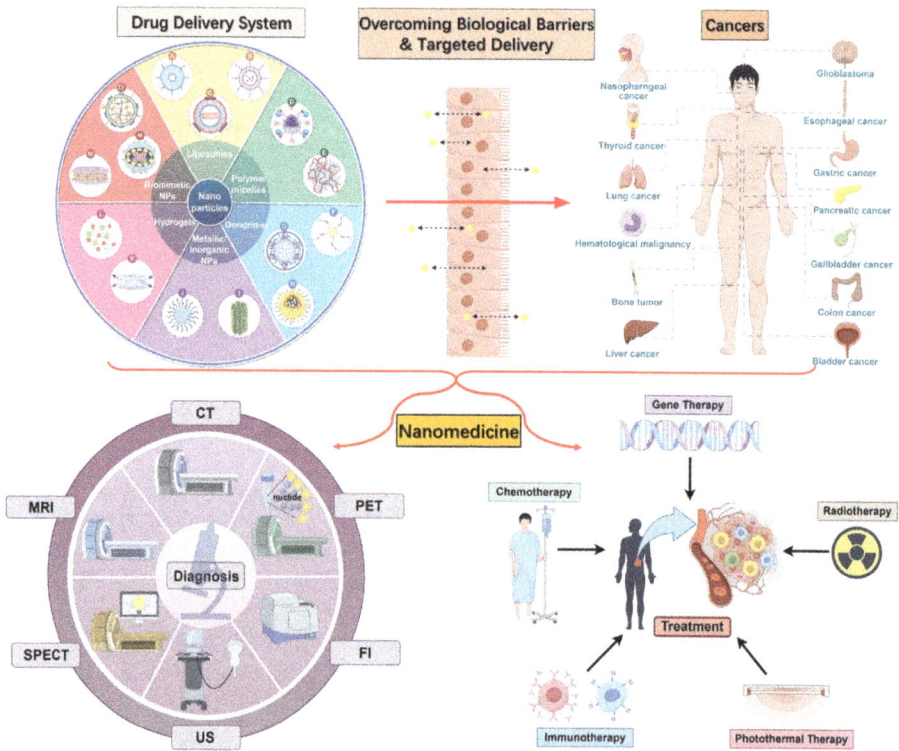

**Fig. 7.2** Role of nanomedicine in cancer diagnosis and treatment [95]

## 7.3 Conclusion

significant limitations, including low absorption through gastrointestinal tract and poor distribution in the target organs. With size ranging from 10 to 800 nm, nanocrystals have a greater surface area that increase the dissolution property of the drugs in the blood, offering higher distribution and bioavailability to promote enhanced biological effect. It is important to note that the biological activity of a drug depends greatly on the particle size, texture and shape. Particles with too small size have higher rate of dissolution, leading to fast excretion, whereas larger particles render easy detection by cells of the Reticular Endothelial System (RES), causing higher accumulation of the nanocrystals in these cells. Nanocrystals can be manufactured both by top-down and bottom-up approaches. While top-down approach starts from bulk material, reducing it to nano level through various processes like ball milling etc., it becomes difficult to control the particle size and shape with high precision. As a result, manufacture of nanocrystals for theranostic purpose at industrial scale appears a major challenge, since commercialized products demand uniformity in particle morphology. On the other hand, bottom-up techniques operate through atoms and molecules as starting material, allowing stringent control on the parameters that can result in uniform nanocrystals that can have greater market acceptance. Therefore, detailed understanding of the nanocrystal behaviour is required in order to develop nanomedicines to meet the specific needs of the patient population.

This book provides a comprehensive understanding about the various types of nanocrystals and their application in cancer theranostics. Nanocrystals can be organic, inorganic as well as hybrid in nature. Organic nanocrystals are biocompatible, show higher tissue penetration capacity and offer less toxicity as they are biodegradable. Inorganic nanocrystals, on the other hand, provide greater surface area and high drug-loading capacity. Hybrid nanocrystals are gaining more popularity nowadays as different drug molecules are combined with agents that enhance the physical and biological property of the crystals. Nanocrystals can act as excellent vehicles for drug delivery and is widely exploited to deliver various anti-cancer agents. Nanocrystals engineered with ligands that recognize cancer cells are exploited to enable targeted therapy at specific cancer microenvironment. They can facilitate immunomodulation and immunotherapy in cancer management. Owing to their small size and high surface area, nanocrystals can act as adjuvants for immunomodulatory drugs, that can activate the T cells, Natural Killer cells and macrophages against tumour cells, and B cells for antibody production. Biotherapeutics like proteins, nucleic acids etc. are often conjugated with nanocrystals to prevent their degradation by enzymatic activity in the body, thus increasing their half-life. Light-reactive nanocrystals have opened a new area of cancer eradication through photodynamic (PTD) and photothermal (PTT) therapy. Recent years have explored plasmonic nanocrystals of gold and silver, carbon-based nanoparticles to generate heat mediated photothermal therapy. In PTD, photosensitive nanocrystals are made to generate ROS through light eradiation to kill the cancer cells. However, much care is needed to be taken to ensure that these therapies are highly target-specific, because they carry high chances of off-site toxicity in the body if not properly controlled.

Biotoxicity is important concern for the success of nanocrystals in cancer theranostics. Research all over the world are generating novel nanomaterials for cancer detection and therapy. Majority of the nanosystems demonstrate partial victory in vitro, being specifically hostile towards the cancer cell lines. These researches lack sufficient data supported by pre-clinical and clinical studies to generate hope to implement the nanocrystals on human patients. The interventions either show poor therapeutic efficacy at safe doses, or are poorly tolerated, giving rise to undesired side effects. Patients withdraw themselves from the studies, which are forced to be terminated much before the scheduled time. As a result, the scientists are shifting their focus to create functionalized nanocrystals which can offer high tolerance among human patients. Initially, the concept of nanocrystal revolved around solid colloidal particles that has minimal surface modulation. In the growing years, nanocrystals with modifiable surfaces are being developed to reduce the off-target toxicity. In this context, bioinspired nanoparticles are becoming popular, wherein nanocrystals or theranostic drugs are conjugated with organic and biological or bioderived agents like proteins, polysaccharides, lipids that are far more biocompatible in the living systems as compared to bare nanocrystals.

Nanocrystals provide a patient-friendly platform in the field of theranostics. They eliminate the individual infusion of therapeutic and diagnostic agents into the patient body, reducing the side effects of multiple drug administration. Nanocrystals combine both the therapeutic and diagnostic/imaging agent in a single unit, which can act synergistically to ensure both detection and targeting of cancer cells. This has simplified cancer treatment, setting the platform for placing the patient's comfort at the highest priority. We can conclude that nanocrystals are being actively investigated in cancer research. Sincere efforts in this field will surely bring potent nanomedicines for cancer in the emerging future.

## 7.4 Future Scope

Nanocrystals hold great potential in the application of cancer theranostics. The dual platform combining diagnosis and therapy is highly promising in the field of cancer treatment. As discussed earlier, one of the major limitations of nanocrystals used in theranostic purposes is their toxic effects on biological systems. Besides the biological mechanism of action, future researchers should pay more attention in developing modified or bioinspired nanocrystals that increase the patient safety and support the clinical translation of the products. More research should be conducted to identify molecules and functional moieties whose conjugation would make the nanocrystals safer and tolerable. Nanocrystals often fail to demonstrate the desired therapeutic effect in the clinical setting due to lack of specificity and ability to recognise the cancer cells. This leads to off-target toxicity. Therefore, it is important for the upcoming research to produce nanocrystals that are highly specific and target the cancer cells, without harming the healthy tissues of the body. The biological activity of nanocrystals depends greatly on its morphology and surface properties, which in turn is dependent of the method of preparation and the precursors used in the process. An important factor that affects the nanocrystal property in this context is the choice of stabilizer. Scientists should be careful in choosing the suitable stabilizer that can help to prepare the nanocrystals with the desired size and structure, and which enhances the biocompatibility. Future work should focus on the optimization of the techniques involved in the synthesis of nanocrystals that have uniform shape, offers high biodistribution and has low instances of toxicity, so that they can be easily commercialised in the market. Efforts should be given in the production of skilled technicians who understand the purpose of the manufactured nanocrystals and how their properties need to be tuned based on their application. Nanocrystals can act as excellent immunomodulators that can reprogram the immune system against cancerous cells. This unique property of nanocrystals is not yet adequately explored. More research needs to be done in the development of nanocrystals containing immunomodulatory molecules. A major breakthrough in this area can be the generation of cancer vaccines using nanocrystals loaded with tumour antigens to educate the immune cells for cancer recognition. Being wonderful carrier agents, nanocrystals can encapsulate genes, siRNAs and increase their stability in biological systems. Future work should lay stress in the development of advanced gene therapy methods for cancer therapeutics. In essence, the future of cancer theranostics is not in just identifying the cancer, but in providing acceptable interventions to manage it, while paving the path to personalized and triumphant patient outcomes.

## References

1. Paris, J. L., Villaverde, G., Gómez-Graña, S., & Vallet-Regí, M. (2020). Nanoparticles for multimodal antivascular therapeutics: Dual drug release, photothermal and photodynamic therapy. *Acta biomaterialia, 101*, 459–468.
2. Mukherjee, A., Waters, A. K., Kalyan, P., Achrol, A. S., Kesari, S., & Yenugonda, V. M. (2019). Lipid–polymer hybrid nanoparticles as a next-generation drug delivery platform: state of the art, emerging technologies, and perspectives. *International journal of nanomedicine*, 1937–1952.
3. Mukherjee, A., Waters, A. K., Babic, I., Nurmemmedov, E., Glassy, M. C., Kesari, S., et al. (2019). Antibody drug conjugates: Progress, pitfalls, and promises. *Human antibodies, 27*(1), 53–62.
4. Kashyap, B. K., Singh, V. V., Solanki, M. K., Kumar, A., Ruokolainen, J., & Kesari, K. K. (2023). Smart nanomaterials in cancer theranostics: challenges and opportunities. *ACS omega, 8*(16), 14290–14320.
5. Yazbeck, V., Alesi, E., Myers, J., Hackney, M. H., Cuttino, L., & Gewirtz, D. A. (2022). An overview of chemotoxicity and radiation toxicity in cancer therapy. *Advances in Cancer Research, 155*, 1–27.
6. Loureiro, A., G. Azoia, N., C. Gomes, A., & Cavaco-Paulo, A. (2016). Albumin-based nanodevices as drug carriers. *Current pharmaceutical design, 22*(10), 1371–1390.
7. Di, J., Gao, X., Du, Y., Zhang, H., Gao, J., & Zheng, A. (2021). Size, shape, charge and "stealthy" surface: Carrier properties affect the drug circulation time in vivo. *Asian journal of pharmaceutical sciences, 16*(4), 444–458.

8. Güven, E. (2021). Nanoparticles for anticancer drug delivery. In *Nanotechnology Applications in Health and Environmental Sciences* (pp. 71–81): Springer.
9. Bruce, J. Y., Eickhoff, J., Pili, R., Logan, T., Carducci, M., Arnott, J., et al. (2012). A phase II study of 2-methoxyestradiol nanocrystal colloidal dispersion alone and in combination with sunitinib malate in patients with metastatic renal cell carcinoma progressing on sunitinib malate. *Investigational new drugs, 30*, 794–802.
10. Racca, L., Rosso, G., Carofiglio, M., Fagoonee, S., Mesiano, G., Altruda, F., et al. (2023). Effective combination of biocompatible zinc oxide nanocrystals and high-energy shock waves for the treatment of colorectal cancer. *Cancer Nanotechnology, 14*(1), 37.
11. Sannino, D. (2021). Types and classification of nanomaterials. *Nanotechnology: Trends and Future Applications*, 15–38.
12. Rashid[1], E. U., Nawaz, S., & Munawar, J. (2022). Organic and inorganic. *Smart Polymer Nanocomposites: Design, Synthesis, Functionalization, Properties, and Applications*, 93.
13. Alwattar, J. K., Mneimneh, A. T., Abla, K. K., Mehanna, M. M., & Allam, A. N. (2021). Smart stimuli-responsive liposomal nanohybrid systems: A critical review of theranostic behavior in cancer. *Pharmaceutics, 13*(3), 355.
14. Hsu, J. C., Tang, Z., Eremina, O. E., Sofias, A. M., Lammers, T., Lovell, J. F., et al. (2023). Nanomaterial-based contrast agents. *Nature Reviews Methods Primers, 3*(1), 30.
15. Exner, A. A., & Kolios, M. C. (2021). Bursting microbubbles: How nanobubble contrast agents can enable the future of medical ultrasound molecular imaging and image-guided therapy. *Current opinion in colloid & interface science, 54*, 101463.
16. Kumari, B., & Prakash, A. (2023). Lipid-based nanoparticles as drug delivery agents. In *Nanoparticles in diagnosis, drug delivery and nanotherapeutics* (pp. 127–149): CRC Press.
17. Lamichhane, N., Udayakumar, T. S., D'Souza, W. D., Simone, C. B., Raghavan, S. R., Polf, J., et al. (2018). Liposomes: clinical applications and potential for image-guided drug delivery. *Molecules, 23*(2), 288.
18. Pattni, B. S., Chupin, V. V., & Torchilin, V. P. (2015). New developments in liposomal drug delivery. *Chemical Reviews, 115*(19), 10938–10966.
19. Wang, J., Zhang, Y., Liu, C., Zha, W., Dong, S., Xing, H., et al. (2022). Multifunctional lipid nanoparticles for protein kinase N3 shRNA delivery and prostate cancer therapy. *Molecular Pharmaceutics, 19*(12), 4588–4600.
20. Liang, X., Chen, M., Bhattarai, P., Hameed, S., Tang, Y., & Dai, Z. (2021). Complementing cancer photodynamic therapy with ferroptosis through iron oxide loaded porphyrin-grafted lipid nanoparticles. *ACS nano, 15*(12), 20164–20180.
21. Wu, G., Hui, X., Hu, L., Bai, Y., Rahaman, A., Yang, X.-F., et al. (2022). Recent advancement of bioinspired nanomaterials and their applications: A review. *Frontiers in Bioengineering and Biotechnology, 10*, 952523.
22. Ni, Q., Zhang, F., Zhang, Y., Zhu, G., Wang, Z., Teng, Z., et al. (2018). In situ shRNA synthesis on DNA–polylactide nanoparticles to treat multidrug resistant breast cancer. *Advanced Materials, 30*(10), 1705737.
23. De France, K. J., Chan, K. J., Cranston, E. D., & Hoare, T. (2016). Enhanced mechanical properties in cellulose nanocrystal–poly (oligoethylene glycol methacrylate) injectable nanocomposite hydrogels through control of physical and chemical cross-linking. *Biomacromolecules, 17*(2), 649–660.
24. Sunasee, R., Hemraz, U. D., & Ckless, K. (2016). Cellulose nanocrystals: A versatile nanoplatform for emerging biomedical applications. *Expert opinion on drug delivery, 13*(9), 1243–1256.
25. Menas, A. L., Yanamala, N., Farcas, M. T., Russo, M., Friend, S., Fournier, P. M., et al. (2017). Fibrillar vs crystalline nanocellulose pulmonary epithelial cell responses: Cytotoxicity or inflammation? *Chemosphere, 171*, 671–680.

26. Imlimthan, S., Khng, Y. C., Keinänen, O., Zhang, W., Airaksinen, A. J., Kostiainen, M. A., et al. (2021). A theranostic cellulose nanocrystal-based drug delivery system with enhanced retention in pulmonary metastasis of melanoma. *Small, 17*(18), 2007705.
27. Ventura, C., Pinto, F., Lourenço, A. F., Ferreira, P. J., Louro, H., & Silva, M. J. (2020). On the toxicity of cellulose nanocrystals and nanofibrils in animal and cellular models. *Cellulose, 27*, 5509–5544.
28. Gradishar, W. J. (2006). Albumin-bound paclitaxel: a next-generation taxane. *Expert opinion on pharmacotherapy, 7*(8), 1041–1053.
29. Safaei, M., Foroughi, M. M., Ebrahimpoor, N., Jahani, S., Omidi, A., & Khatami, M. (2019). A review on metal-organic frameworks: Synthesis and applications. *TrAC Trends in Analytical Chemistry, 118*, 401–425.
30. Γκιλιόπουλος, Δ., Ζαμπούλη, Α., Γιαννακουδάκης, Δ., Μπικιάρης, Δ., & Τριανταφυλλίδης, Κ. (2020). Polymer/metal organic framework (MOF) nanocomposites for biomedical applications.
31. Chen, Y., Zhong, H., Wang, J., Wan, X., Li, Y., Pan, W., et al. (2019). Catalase-like metal–organic framework nanoparticles to enhance radiotherapy in hypoxic cancer and prevent cancer recurrence. *Chemical Science, 10*(22), 5773–5778.
32. Ren, Q., Yu, N., Wang, L., Wen, M., Geng, P., Jiang, Q., et al. (2022). Nanoarchitectonics with metal-organic frameworks and platinum nanozymes with improved oxygen evolution for enhanced sonodynamic/chemo-therapy. *Journal of Colloid and Interface Science, 614*, 147–159.
33. Zhu, W., Yang, Y., Jin, Q., Chao, Y., Tian, L., Liu, J., et al. (2019). Two-dimensional metal-organic-framework as a unique theranostic nano-platform for nuclear imaging and chemo-photodynamic cancer therapy. *Nano Research, 12*, 1307–1312.
34. Ahmadi, M., Ayyoubzadeh, S. M., Ghorbani-Bidkorbeh, F., Shahhosseini, S., Dadashzadeh, S., Asadian, E., et al. (2021). An investigation of affecting factors on MOF characteristics for biomedical applications: A systematic review. *Heliyon, 7*(4).
35. Gao, X., Zhai, M., Guan, W., Liu, J., Liu, Z., & Damirin, A. (2017). Controllable synthesis of a smart multifunctional nanoscale metal–organic framework for magnetic resonance/optical imaging and targeted drug delivery. *ACS Applied Materials & Interfaces, 9*(4), 3455–3462.
36. Gao, X., Cui, R., Ji, G., & Liu, Z. (2018). Size and surface controllable metal–organic frameworks (MOFs) for fluorescence imaging and cancer therapy. *Nanoscale, 10*(13), 6205–6211.
37. Cherkasov, V. R., Mochalova, E. N., Babenyshev, A. V., Rozenberg, J. M., Sokolov, I. L., & Nikitin, M. P. (2020). Antibody-directed metal-organic framework nanoparticles for targeted drug delivery. *Acta biomaterialia, 103*, 223–236.
38. Chen, L., & Liang, J. (2020). An overview of functional nanoparticles as novel emerging antiviral therapeutic agents. *Materials Science and Engineering: C, 112*, 110924.
39. Caiyan, Y., Tongtong, X., Sunqi, L., Xiaoxiao, L., Guohai, L., & Huili, L. (2017). Gd3+ doped CuInS2/ZnS nanocrystals with high quantum yield for bimodal fluorescence/magnetic resonance imaging. *Journal of Rare Earths, 35*(4), 382–388.
40. Zayed, D. G., AbdElhamid, A. S., Freag, M. S., & Elzoghby, A. O. (2019). Hybrid quantum dot-based theranostic nanomedicines for tumor-targeted drug delivery and cancer imaging. (Vol. 14, pp. 225–228): Taylor & Francis.
41. De la Cruz, G. G., Rodríguez-Fragoso, L., Rodríguez-Fragoso, P., & Rodríguez-López, A. (2024). Toxicity of quantum dots. In *Toxicity of Nanoparticles-Recent Advances and New Perspectives*: IntechOpen.
42. Chen, H., Liu, Z., Wei, B., Huang, J., You, X., Zhang, J., et al. (2021). Redox responsive nanoparticle encapsulating black phosphorus quantum dots for cancer theranostics. *Bioactive materials, 6*(3), 655–665.
43. Filali, S., Pirot, F., & Miossec, P. (2020). Biological applications and toxicity minimization of semiconductor quantum dots. *Trends in biotechnology, 38*(2), 163-177.

44. Aguilar-Pérez, K., Avilés-Castrillo, J., Ruiz-Pulido, G., Medina, D. I., Parra-Saldivar, R., & Iqbal, H. M. (2021). Nanoadsorbents in focus for the remediation of environmentally-related contaminants with rising toxicity concerns. *Science of The Total Environment, 779*, 146465.
45. He, K., Hu, C., Ding, Y.-F., Cai, W., Huang, D., Mo, L., et al. (2024). Renal-clearable luminescent gold nanoparticles incorporating active and bio-orthogonal tumor-targeting for drug delivery and controlled release. *Nano Today, 56*, 102245.
46. Wang, Z.-G., Liu, S.-L., & Pang, D.-W. (2021). Quantum dots: a promising fluorescent label for probing virus trafficking. *Accounts of chemical research, 54*(14), 2991–3002.
47. Vaishanav, S. K., Korram, J., Nagwanshi, R., Karbhal, I., Dewangan, L., Ghosh, K. K., et al. (2021). Interaction of Folic Acid with Mn 2+ Doped CdTe/ZnS Quantum Dots: In Situ Detection of Folic Acid. *Journal of Fluorescence, 31*, 951–960.
48. Chong, Y., Ma, Y., Shen, H., Tu, X., Zhou, X., Xu, J., et al. (2014). The in vitro and in vivo toxicity of graphene quantum dots. *Biomaterials, 35*(19), 5041–5048.
49. Yadav, S., Singh Raman, A. P., Meena, H., Goswami, A. G., Bhawna, Kumar, V., et al. (2022). An update on graphene oxide: applications and toxicity. *ACS omega, 7*(40), 35387–35445.
50. Xue, X., Li, J., Chen, T., Cui, M., Liang, H., Zhang, Y., et al. (2025). Molecularly Engineered NIR-II Emitting Carbon Dots Assemblies for Unprecedented High-Resolution Angiography and Synergistic Photodynamic/Photothermal Tumor Therapy. *Chemical Engineering Journal, 505*, 159356.
51. Zhi, B., Yao, X., Cui, Y., Orr, G., & Haynes, C. L. (2019). Synthesis, applications and potential photoluminescence mechanism of spectrally tunable carbon dots. *Nanoscale, 11*(43), 20411–20428.
52. Zhang, L., Lin, Z., Yu, Y.-X., Jiang, B.-P., & Shen, X.-C. (2018). Multifunctional hyaluronic acid-derived carbon dots for self-targeted imaging-guided photodynamic therapy. *Journal of Materials Chemistry B, 6*(41), 6534–6543.
53. Tasnim, K. N., Adrita, S. H., Hossain, S., Akash, S. Z., & Sharker, S. (2020). The prospect of stem cells for HIV and cancer treatment: a review. *Pharmaceutical and Biomedical Research*.
54. Lin, C., Sun, K., Zhang, C., Tan, T., Xu, M., Liu, Y., et al. (2020). Carbon dots embedded metal organic framework@ chitosan core-shell nanoparticles for vitro dual mode imaging and pH-responsive drug delivery. *Microporous and Mesoporous Materials, 293*, 109775.
55. Zhang, Z., Lei, Y., Yang, X., Shi, N., Geng, L., Wang, S., et al. (2019). High drug-loading system of hollow carbon dots–doxorubicin: Preparation, in vitro release and pH-targeted research. *Journal of Materials Chemistry B, 7*(13), 2130–2137.
56. Jia, Q., Zhao, Z., Liang, K., Nan, F., Li, Y., Wang, J., et al. (2020). Recent advances and prospects of carbon dots in cancer nanotheranostics. *Materials Chemistry Frontiers, 4*(2), 449–471.
57. Yang, W., Wei, B., Yang, Z., & Sheng, L. (2019). Facile synthesis of novel carbon-dots/hemin nanoplatforms for synergistic photo-thermal and photo-dynamic therapies. *Journal of Inorganic Biochemistry, 193*, 166–172.
58. Chen, J., Fan, T., Xie, Z., Zeng, Q., Xue, P., Zheng, T., et al. (2020). Advances in nanomaterials for photodynamic therapy applications: Status and challenges. *Biomaterials, 237*, 119827.
59. Shi, H., Gu, R., Xu, W., Huang, H., Xue, L., Wang, W., et al. (2019). Near-infrared light-harvesting fullerene-based nanoparticles for promoted synergetic tumor phototheranostics. *ACS Applied Materials & Interfaces, 11*(48), 44970–44977.
60. Wang, T., & Wang, C. (2019). Functional metallofullerene materials and their applications in nanomedicine, magnetics, and electronics. *Small, 15*(48), 1901522.
61. Ye, L., Kollie, L., Liu, X., Guo, W., Ying, X., Zhu, J., et al. (2021). Antitumor activity and potential mechanism of novel fullerene derivative nanoparticles. *Molecules, 26*(11), 3252.

62. Serda, M., Ware, M. J., Newton, J. M., Sachdeva, S., Krzykawska-Serda, M., Nguyen, L., et al. (2018). Development of photoactive Sweet-C60 for pancreatic cancer stellate cell therapy. *Nanomedicine, 13*(23), 2981–2993.
63. Mostafavi, E., & Zare, H. (2022). Carbon-based nanomaterials in gene therapy. *OpenNano, 7*, 100062.
64. Zhou, H., Ge, J., Miao, Q., Zhu, R., Wen, L., Zeng, J., et al. (2019). Biodegradable inorganic nanoparticles for cancer theranostics: Insights into the degradation behavior. *Bioconjugate chemistry, 31*(2), 315–331.
65. Park, Y., Yoo, J., Kang, M.-H., Kwon, W., & Joo, J. (2019). Photoluminescent and biodegradable porous silicon nanoparticles for biomedical imaging. *Journal of Materials Chemistry B, 7*(41), 6271–6292.
66. Thapa, R., Ali, H., Afzal, O., Bhat, A. A., Almalki, W. H., Alzarea, S. I., et al. (2023). Unlocking the potential of mesoporous silica nanoparticles in breast cancer treatment. *Journal of Nanoparticle Research, 25*(8), 169.
67. Shakeran, Z., Keyhanfar, M., Varshosaz, J., & Sutherland, D. S. (2021). Biodegradable nanocarriers based on chitosan-modified mesoporous silica nanoparticles for delivery of methotrexate for application in breast cancer treatment. *Materials Science and Engineering: C, 118*, 111526.
68. Gu, L., Fang, R. H., Sailor, M. J., & Park, J.-H. (2012). In vivo clearance and toxicity of monodisperse iron oxide nanocrystals. *ACS nano, 6*(6), 4947–4954.
69. Iravani, S., Korbekandi, H., Mirmohammadi, S. V., & Zolfaghari, B. (2014). Synthesis of silver nanoparticles: chemical, physical and biological methods. *Research in pharmaceutical sciences, 9*(6), 385–406.
70. Ferdous, Z., & Nemmar, A. (2020). Health impact of silver nanoparticles: a review of the biodistribution and toxicity following various routes of exposure. *International journal of molecular sciences, 21*(7), 2375.
71. Loza, K., Diendorf, J., Sengstock, C., Ruiz-Gonzalez, L., Gonzalez-Calbet, J., Vallet-Regi, M., et al. (2014). The dissolution and biological effects of silver nanoparticles in biological media. *Journal of Materials Chemistry B, 2*(12), 1634–1643.
72. Padinjarathil, H., Joseph, M. M., Unnikrishnan, B., Preethi, G., Shiji, R., Archana, M., et al. (2018). Galactomannan endowed biogenic silver nanoparticles exposed enhanced cancer cytotoxicity with excellent biocompatibility. *International journal of biological macromolecules, 118*, 1174–1182.
73. Oves, M., Aslam, M., Rauf, M. A., Qayyum, S., Qari, H. A., Khan, M. S., et al. (2018). Antimicrobial and anticancer activities of silver nanoparticles synthesized from the root hair extract of Phoenix dactylifera. *Materials Science and Engineering: C, 89*, 429–443.
74. Maity, P., Bepari, M., Pradhan, A., Baral, R., Roy, S., & Choudhury, S. M. (2018). Synthesis and characterization of biogenic metal nanoparticles and its cytotoxicity and anti-neoplasticity through the induction of oxidative stress, mitochondrial dysfunction and apoptosis. *Colloids and Surfaces B: Biointerfaces, 161*, 111–120.
75. Dinparvar, S., Bagirova, M., Allahverdiyev, A. M., Abamor, E. S., Safarov, T., Aydogdu, M., et al. (2020). A nanotechnology-based new approach in the treatment of breast cancer: Biosynthesized silver nanoparticles using Cuminum cyminum L. seed extract. *Journal of Photochemistry and Photobiology B: Biology, 208*, 111902.
76. Chu, S., & Stochaj, U. (2020). Exploring near-infrared absorbing nanocarriers to overcome cancer drug resistance. *Cancer Drug Resistance, 3*(3), 302.
77. Zhao, Y., Song, M., Yang, X., Yang, J., Du, C., Wang, G., et al. (2020). Amorphous $Ag_{2-x}Cu_xS$ quantum dots: "all-in-one" theranostic nanomedicines for near-infrared fluorescence/photoacoustics dual-modal-imaging-guided photothermal therapy. *Chemical Engineering Journal, 399*, 125777.

78. Yun, Y., Kim, S., Lee, S.-N., Cho, H.-Y., & Choi, J.-W. (2024). Nanomaterial-based detection of circulating tumor cells and circulating cancer stem cells for cancer immunotherapy. *Nano Convergence, 11*(1), 1–27.
79. Matei, D., Schilder, J., Sutton, G., Perkins, S., Breen, T., Quon, C., et al. (2009). Activity of 2 methoxyestradiol (Panzem® NCD) in advanced, platinum-resistant ovarian cancer and primary peritoneal carcinomatosis: A hoosier oncology group trial. *Gynecologic oncology, 115*(1), 90–96.
80. Sweeney, C., Liu, G., Yiannoutsos, C., Kolesar, J., Horvath, D., Staab, M. J., et al. (2005). A phase II multicenter, randomized, double-blind, safety trial assessing the pharmacokinetics, pharmacodynamics, and efficacy of oral 2-methoxyestradiol capsules in hormone-refractory prostate cancer. *Clinical cancer research, 11*(18), 6625–6633.
81. Atkins, M. B., Redman, B., Mier, J., Gollob, J., Weber, J., Sosman, J., et al. (2001). A phase I study of CNI-1493, an inhibitor of cytokine release, in combination with high-dose interleukin-2 in patients with renal cancer and melanoma. *Clinical cancer research, 7*(3), 486–492.
82. Guo, S., & Huang, L. (2014). Nanoparticles containing insoluble drug for cancer therapy. *Biotechnology advances, 32*(4), 778–788.
83. Robins, D. J., Sui, W., Matulay, J. T., Ghandour, R., Anderson, C. B., DeCastro, G. J., et al. (2017). Long-term survival outcomes with intravesical nanoparticle albumin-bound paclitaxel for recurrent non–muscle-invasive bladder cancer after previous bacillus Calmette-Guérin therapy. *Urology, 103*, 149–153.
84. Gradishar, W. J., Tjulandin, S., Davidson, N., Shaw, H., Desai, N., Bhar, P., et al. (2005). Phase III trial of nanoparticle albumin-bound paclitaxel compared with polyethylated castor oil-based paclitaxel in women with breast cancer. *J Clin Oncol, 23*(31), 7794–7803, https://doi.org/10.1200/jco.2005.04.937.
85. Li, X., Ferrel, G. L., Guerra, M. C., Hode, T., Lunn, J. A., Adalsteinsson, O., et al. (2011). Preliminary safety and efficacy results of laser immunotherapy for the treatment of metastatic breast cancer patients. *Photochemical & Photobiological Sciences, 10*(5), 817–821, https://doi.org/10.1039/C0PP00306A.
86. Senzer, N. N., Matsuno, K., Yamagata, N., Fujisawa, T., Wasserman, E., Sutherland, W., et al. (2009). Abstract C36: MBP-426, a novel liposome-encapsulated oxaliplatin, in combination with 5-FU/leucovorin (LV): Phase I results of a Phase I/II study in gastro-esophageal adenocarcinoma, with pharmacokinetics. *Molecular Cancer Therapeutics, 8*(12_Supplement), C36–C36, https://doi.org/10.1158/1535-7163.targ-09-c36.
87. Zhang, R., Kiessling, F., Lammers, T., & Pallares, R. M. (2023). Clinical translation of gold nanoparticles. *Drug Delivery and Translational Research, 13*(2), 378–385, https://doi.org/10.1007/s13346-022-01232-4.
88. Phillips, E., Penate-Medina, O., Zanzonico, P. B., Carvajal, R. D., Mohan, P., Ye, Y., et al. (2014). Clinical translation of an ultrasmall inorganic optical-PET imaging nanoparticle probe. *Science Translational Medicine, 6*(260), 260ra149–260ra149, https://doi.org/10.1126/scitranslmed.3009524.
89. Autio, K. A., Dreicer, R., Anderson, J., Garcia, J. A., Alva, A., Hart, L. L., et al. (2018). Safety and Efficacy of BIND-014, a Docetaxel Nanoparticle Targeting Prostate-Specific Membrane Antigen for Patients With Metastatic Castration-Resistant Prostate Cancer: A Phase 2 Clinical Trial. *JAMA Oncology, 4*(10), 1344–1351, https://doi.org/10.1001/jamaoncol.2018.2168.
90. Boere, I., Vergote, I., Hanssen, R., Jalving, M., Gennigens, C., Ottevanger, P., et al. (2023). CINOVA: a phase II study of CPC634 (nanoparticulate docetaxel) in patients with platinum resistant recurrent ovarian cancer. *International Journal of Gynecological Cancer, 33*(8), 1247–1252, https://doi.org/10.1136/ijgc-2023-004308.

91. El Dika, I., Lim, H. Y., Yong, W. P., Lin, C. C., Yoon, J. H., Modiano, M., et al. (2019). An open-label, multicenter, phase I, dose escalation study with phase II expansion cohort to determine the safety, pharmacokinetics, and preliminary antitumor activity of intravenous TKM-080301 in subjects with advanced hepatocellular carcinoma. *The oncologist, 24*(6), 747-e218.
92. Schmidt, K. T., Peer, C. J., Huitema, A. D., Williams, M. D., Wroblewski, S., Schellens, J. H., et al. (2020). Measurement of NLG207 (formerly CRLX101) nanoparticle-bound and released camptothecin in human plasma. *Journal of pharmaceutical and biomedical analysis, 181*, 113073.
93. Thivat, E., Casile, M., Moreau, J., Molnar, I., Dufort, S., Seddik, K., et al. (2023). Phase I/II study testing the combination of AGuIX nanoparticles with radiochemotherapy and concomitant temozolomide in patients with newly diagnosed glioblastoma (NANO-GBM trial protocol). *BMC cancer, 23*(1), 344.
94. Bonvalot, S., Rutkowski, P. L., Thariat, J., Carrère, S., Ducassou, A., Sunyach, M.-P., et al. (2019). NBTXR3, a first-in-class radioenhancer hafnium oxide nanoparticle, plus radiotherapy versus radiotherapy alone in patients with locally advanced soft-tissue sarcoma (Act. In. Sarc): a multicentre, phase 2–3, randomised, controlled trial. *The Lancet Oncology, 20*(8), 1148–1159.
95. Wang, B., Hu, S., Teng, Y., Chen, J., Wang, H., Xu, Y., et al. (2024). Current advance of nanotechnology in diagnosis and treatment for malignant tumors. *Signal Transduction and Targeted Therapy, 9*(1), 200, https://doi.org/10.1038/s41392-024-01889-y.

GPSR Compliance

The European Union's (EU) General Product Safety Regulation (GPSR) is a set of rules that requires consumer products to be safe and our obligations to ensure this.

If you have any concerns about our products, you can contact us on

ProductSafety@springernature.com

In case Publisher is established outside the EU, the EU authorized representative is:

Springer Nature Customer Service Center GmbH
Europaplatz 3
69115 Heidelberg, Germany

www.ingramcontent.com/pod-product-compliance
Lightning Source LLC
Chambersburg PA
CBHW081711031125
34911CB00003B/87